"I found myself cheering the perceptiveness and humanity that shone out of the book. It is easy to be sympathetic to handicapped children; it's not so easy to be practical and sensible at the same time, and to deal with the conflicting schools of thought with fairness and with the humility born of the knowledge that people are trying their best in a difficult situation. Nowhere is this more clearly shown than in the way the authors deal with parents of deaf children. These parents have, in many previous books, been part of the "Blame the Victim" theory of education. The writers never did this. Bless them for not doing it. And bless them, too, for the clarity and skillfulness of the writing itself. As a writer, I was moved by the amount of information, both medical and psychological, that they were able to convey in what seemed to me to be a very short book. I don't want to say this is a small book because I think it is a very big book, and will remain so for many years."

Joanne Greenberg
Author of *I Never Promised You a Rose Garden* and of *In This Sign*

"The book is excellent. I think it will quickly become the leading guide for parents of deaf children (as well as professionals who work with them)."

Thomas S. Spradley
Co-author of *Deaf Like Me*

"In my view it is the most realistic approach to the problems of the deaf child and his family. It should be read by the parents of every hearing handicapped child and by all of those in education who have any responsibility for planning programs for the hearing impaired or counseling the families of deaf children.

It should also be read by members of the medical profession, particularly otologists and pediatricians, who so often are the first professionals to counsel the parents of deaf children after a child's hearing loss has been diagnosed."

Richard G. Brill, Ed.D.
Retired Superintendent
California School for the Deaf, Riverside

"The book appears to me to respond to the mission of the authors admirably. As a guide, it is written from the point of view of parents and those who work with deaf children. It is almost a step by step identification of the issues which these persons will face, an analysis of these issues, and a point of view or a position which is definitely child-centered. I admire the candid, sound advice which appears. Parents are not talked down to nor are they patronized. The book is trying to be practical and realistic with parents. The book will permit parents of deaf children and those who work with them to assist them to grow into young people who can capitalize on their potential and have a good feeling about themselves regardless of their hearing impairment."

Edward C. Merrill, Jr.
President, Gallaudet College

"This book is a must for parents who want only the best for their deaf children."

Leo M. Jacobs
Author of *A Deaf Adult Speaks Out*

CAN'T YOUR CHILD HEAR?
A Guide for Those Who Care about Deaf Children

by

Roger D. Freeman, M.D.
Professor
Department of Psychiatry
University of British Columbia
Vancouver, B.C.

Clifton F. Carbin, M.Ed.
Director
Counselling and Home Training Program for Deaf Children
Children's Hospital Diagnostic Centre
Vancouver, B.C.

Robert J. Boese, Ph.D.
Clinical Associate Professor
Department of Paediatrics (Medical Sociology)
University of British Columbia
Vancouver, B.C.

Sponsored by:
The International Association of Parents of the Deaf

UNIVERSITY PARK PRESS
Baltimore

UNIVERSITY PARK PRESS
International Publishers in Science, Medicine, and Education
300 North Charles Street
Baltimore, Maryland 21201

Typeset by Maryland Composition Company, Inc.
Manufactured in the United States of America
by The Maple Press Company

Cover   Clifton and Sandi Carbin with their deaf daughter
Carley. Photograph taken by Ian Lindsay.
Reprinted here by permission of The Vancouver Sun.

Acknowledgments   Excerpt from Dorothy Miles, p. *125*, is used with
permission of publisher. Taken from *Gestures* by Dorothy Miles © Joyce
Motion Picture Company, 1976, Northridge, California. Excerpts from
Susan Gregory, *The Deaf Child and His Family*, reprinted here by
permission of publisher © Allen & Unwin, 1976, London. Figure 1,
"Structure of the Ear," appears by permission of Philips Electronics,
Ltd. Figures 2 through 5, sample audiograms, provided by George
Muller. Photograph of Gallaudet College, Figure 10, courtesy of Charles
Shoup and Gallaudet College. Figures 11 and 12, illustrating TDDs and
Message Center, provided by Gordon J. K. Gell and Children's
Hospital, through the Western Institute for the Deaf.

Library of Congress Cataloging in Publication Data

Freeman, Roger D.
  Can't your child hear?

  Bibliography: p.
  Includes index.
  1. Children, Deaf.   2. Children, Deaf—Family
relationships.   3. Deaf—Education.   I. Carbin,
Clifton F.   II. Boese, Robert J.   III. International
Association of Parents of the Deaf.   IV. Title.
  [DNLM: 1. Deafness—In infancy and childhood—Popular
works. WV 271 F855c]
  HV2391.F73   362.4'2'088054   81-4993
  ISBN 0-8391-1616-0   AACR2

Contents

Foreword

Can't Your Child Hear? is a comprehensive resource summarizing and digesting evidence, opinions, and experiences. It recognizes the basic desire of parents—to learn how best to raise healthy, happy children—and points toward wise choices based on fact.

Members of the Executive Board of the International Association of Parents of the Deaf immediately endorsed this approach when the authors first sought our assistance. We know from our own experience and from talking to other parents that families of deaf children around the world need and want reliable, realistic information.

It is impossible to raise a deaf child without considering ways to communicate with that child. Conflicting advice from doctors, audiologists, teachers, and others who first provide care to the child and family complicates important issues: How can a deaf child be raised to fully participate in family life, and be adequately prepared for formal education? How can the deaf child grow to become an independent member of society?

There are differences of opinion about *how* to communicate, but there is general agreement that early, meaningful communication is the key to life for all children. Without question, the most serious obstacle deaf children face is not the lack of hearing, but the difficulty involved in developing an adequate communication system.

The focus of this guide is Total Communication as a way of life for deaf children, their families, their schools, and their communities. As defined here, Total Communication is a flexible, individualized approach based on the skills and needs of each deaf child.

The majority of school programs for deaf children across the United States has now adopted the Total Communication approach. Parents often wonder how effective these classes are. The section "How Can You Judge the Adequacy of a Total Communication Program?" (found in the Total Communication chapter of this guide) will be of great assistance to parents and to all concerned with quality education.

The amount of information collected here is vast. Each person reading this guide will take from it according to his or her needs, and these needs will change from time to time. Chapter headings span concerns of parents throughout a deaf child's life. Concise summaries at the end of each chapter serve as refresher courses, or perhaps as introductions, to the questions involved.

I hope that each parent reading this book will know the same kind of joy that I have known in raising a daughter who is deaf. The days have not all been easy; the nights have not all been peaceful; the decisions have not always been correct. The things that I would change if I could go back 16 years might have been avoidable if I had had a guide such as *Can't Your Child Hear?*

Bonnie Fairchild
President
International Association of Parents of the Deaf

Preface

In the past few years there has been an explosion of new ideas and developments in the field of deafness. Concepts about education and services are changing. So quick has this change been that few parents or non-specialist professional workers are aware of even the most significant developments and their implications. Those working in the area of deafness find it difficult to keep pace with the thinking of their colleagues in other countries and in related fields. We have tried to bring together many sources of information with the belief that informed parents and professionals are essential for the well-being of deaf children. Openness to new ideas and theories is always highly desirable in a rapidly changing field. Many issues are still unresolved; we have tried not to present these as settled if they are not.

For whom is this book intended? Parents of children whose hearing loss is severe or profound, and occurred before the onset of normal speech, are our primary audience. These children are unlikely to be able to depend upon speech, lipreading, and amplification alone. Some of their needs are very different from children known as hard-of-hearing or partially hearing. This book will be less applicable to the latter, and to those who lost their hearing after speech developed. (These children are not less deserving of attention, but we could not include everything in one volume.)

Second, we hope that professional workers in a wide range of fields will find the book useful. It is difficult to write for both parents and professionals, and we may not always have succeeded in striking the correct balance. The references given at the end of the text are both for the general reader and for the specialist. We have found it impossible to designate a sharp dividing line between references that are suitable for one or for the other of these two groups, but nevertheless we have made an attempt to distinguish between them by marking those references that we feel are intended for general readers with an asterisk (*).

Demands of space and readability have limited the thoroughness of referencing. Not every statement or opinion is fully documented. If you want further references, please let us know.

Because of the controversial nature of childhood deafness and its management, as well as rapid developments in other parts of the world, we decided on an unusual procedure. Each chapter in first-draft form was sent to some 60 resource persons (listed in the next section) for comments on clarity of writing, accuracy, and fairness of content, and any other suggestions that they might have. We needed people with different skills and points of view. First and foremost we asked parents to help, because this book is intended primarily for them. In addition to representatives of our sponsor, the International Association of Parents of the Deaf (IAPD), located in Silver Spring, Maryland, and parents known to us personally, we had the assistance of parents from Canada, the United States, the United Kingdom (Great Britain), and Sweden. The second group consisted of deaf people (born deaf and deafened later in life) from several countries. The third group included professionals from every discipline we could think of, and from nine countries (Australia, Canada, Denmark, France, Israel, Malaysia, Sweden, the United Kingdom, and the United States.) The French connection was important not only because of recent developments there, but because of the possibility of an eventual French translation for our own Province of Quebec and other areas of the world linked to French language and culture.

It is fair to say that without the resource persons, the book could not have been completed. They gave unstintingly of their time and effort. As will be seen in the next section, a large proportion of them are prelingually deaf. If anyone has the idea that deaf people who use sign language cannot use good English also, a reading of the comments from these individuals would eliminate that idea!

For the most part, our resource persons assisted only with the first draft and, because of inevitable differences in point of view, they cannot be held responsible for our statements or errors, nor should any blanket endorsement by them of our programs be assumed.

We have often used the second person ("you") to address the reader. This has been done to avoid the awkward language that otherwise results when referring to parents. It is assumed that professionals who are not parents of deaf children will understand.

Because the use of the word *deaf* as a noun is thought by many people to perpetuate the idea that all deaf persons are somehow alike, we have adopted the recent convention of using it only as an adjective, with the exception of its older usage in organizational names or the still-current phrase "teacher of the deaf."

We invite you to provide us with criticisms, comments, and additional information that may be helpful in preparing future editions.

Roger D. Freeman
Clifton F. Carbin
Robert J. Boese

Authors' correspondence address: Counselling and Home Training Program for Deaf Children, Children's Hospital, Vancouver, B.C., Canada V6H 3V4

Acknowledgments

Many people in addition to our resource colleagues made the completion of this book possible.

Dr. David Crockett, Dr. Peter MacLean, Edgar Froese, Derek Allen, and Elizabeth Harmer made it possible to computer-format the chapters for easier editing. The staff of the Western Institute for the Deaf (Gary Magarrell, Lynn Siddaway, Doug Clifton, and Dominique Michel) helped in numerous ways. The teachers at our Bobolink Children's Centre of the Total Communication Children's Society (Sandra Kurbis, Sandy LeMonnier, Susan Weese, and Catherine Welburn) assisted with the chapter on preschools. Dr. Pat Baird, Head, Department of Medical Genetics, University of British Columbia, helped with Chapter 5. Doug Lambert assisted with the photography, but we were not able to utilize his work because of stringent space limitations. Biomedical Communications (University of B.C.) completed most of the art work on the diagrams in a very short time. Thanks are also due A. B. Hayhurst, M.B.E., and A. F. Dimmock for facilitating contact with endorsing organizations in the United Kingdom.

Our thinking about the role of amplification and auditory training was stimulated by discussions with Dr. John Gilbert, Acting Director, School of Audiology and Speech Sciences at the University of British Columbia.

Much of the difficult and detailed administration was capably handled by Toby Moyls and Sharon Rempel.

None of this work would have been possible without the financial assistance of government for the operation of our programs: a demonstration grant from Health and Welfare Canada and support from the Ministries of Education, Health, and Human Resources of the Province of British Columbia.

Support for the Counselling and Home Training Program for Deaf Children was also received from the Vancouver Foundation, the B.C. Ladies' Auxiliary of the Royal Canadian Legion, the Children's Hospital, the Elks Purple Cross Deaf Detection and Development Fund, the Rotary Club of Vancouver (B.C.), the B.C. Lions' Society for Crippled Children (Camp Squamish), and North Vancouver School District 44 (North Vancouver Outdoor School).

Dr. Geoffrey C. Robinson, Professor of Paediatrics (now head of the Division of Population Paediatrics), was instrumental in helping the Counselling and Home Training Program get from the planning to the implementation stage while he was Director of the Children's Hospital Diagnostic Centre.

Finally, the Department of Psychiatry, University of British Columbia, and the Children's Hospital (Vancouver) made completion of the book possible within a very short time. We thank them for their confidence in us. It is also traditional for authors to thank their spouses (Ethel, Sandi, and Marian) and families, and we are no exception. They tolerated phone calls and frequent meetings for over 12 months.

Resource Persons

Note: The following is a list of all those persons who read and commented upon several chapters of this book. We felt it would be of general interest to tell something about them, but obviously much has been omitted. When their place of work or residence is not obvious, it has been indicated in parentheses. (Degrees shown are only those beyond the Bachelor's level, unless they represent special training related to deafness, as in the case of Australia.)

Under *Experience* we have included any close personal relationship with hearing impairment. You may note that nine are prelingually deaf, four are postlingually deafened, and one is severely hard-of-hearing; 18 have prelingually deaf children and one has a postlingually deafened child; five have a deaf spouse; then there are additional overlaps of categories. Thus, 20% are themselves hearing-impaired, and the same proportion are parents of hearing-impaired children.

CANADA

John L. Anderson, M.A., Principal, Saskatchewan School for the Deaf (Saskatoon); National Director, Association of Canadian Educators of the Hearing Impaired. *Training:* special education and education of the deaf. *Experience:* teacher of the deaf; administration.

William Bain, Rehabilitation Counsellor, Western Institute for the Deaf (Vancouver). *Experience:* prelingually deaf; deaf parents and wife.

Kenneth Cambon, M.D., Clinical Associate Professor, Department of Surgery, University of British Columbia; Otologist, Children's Hospital Diagnostic Centre (Vancouver). *Training:* medicine (otology). *Experience:* work with deaf children since 1958.

Lorraine Campbell, Board Member, Total Communication Children's Society (Vancouver). *Experience:* 4-year-old prelingually deaf son.

Bryan R. Clarke, Ph.D., Professor of Educational Psychology and Special Education and Director, Graduate Diploma Program in Education of the Deaf, University of British Columbia (Vancouver). *Training:* psychology, audiology, education. *Experience:* over 25 years experience with deaf children.

Joseph G. Demeza, Superintendent, 1953–79 (retired), Sir James Whitney School for the Deaf (Belleville, Ontario). *Training:* education. *Experience:* member, Executive Committee, Conference of Executives of American Schools for the Deaf and Convention of American Instructors of the Deaf; life member, Board of Directors, Canadian Hearing Society (Toronto): honorary director, Ontario Parents' Council for the Deaf.

Maureen Donald, Retired teacher (1945–78), Jericho Hill School for the Deaf (Vancouver). *Experience:* early onset of profound deafness; directs local TV program "Show of Hands."

Faith Dorman, Past President, Jericho Hill School for the Deaf Parent Society (Surrey, B.C.). *Experience:* mother of 11-year-old prelingually deaf son.

Gordon Fairbank, Founder, Metro Toronto Parents for Total Communication; hearing representative for Ontario Parents' Council on Ontario Co-ordinating Council for the Hearing Impaired; member, Board of Directors, Canadian Hearing Society (Toronto, Ontario). *Experience:* 10-year-old prelingually deaf son.

Henry Minto, M.S., Principal, Jericho Hill School for the Deaf (Vancouver). *Training:* general education, special education, education of the deaf. *Experience:* Executive Director, MacKay Center for Deaf and Crippled Children, Montreal.

Carol Reich, Ph.D., Associate Professor, Department of Special Education, Ontario Institute for Studies in Education (Toronto). *Training:* social psychology. *Experience:* research on preschool deaf children.

Michael Rodda, Ph.D., Professor and Director of Deafness Studies, Department of Educational Psychology, University of Alberta (Edmonton). *Training:* psychology. *Experience:* research on educational outcomes for deaf children in the U.K.

Rev. Robert Rumball, D.D., L.L.D., C.M., Executive Director, Ontario Mission of the Deaf (Toronto). *Training:* ministry. *Experience:* minister for the deaf; community organizer; director of camp, schools, group homes; has 6-year-old adopted prelingually deaf Korean daughter; received Order of Canada for dedicated service to Ontario deaf community.

Christine and Leo Verstraete, Parents of 8-year-old prelingually deaf son (Vancouver). Leo has a brother and sister, both prelingually deaf; Christine was a Registered Nurse.

Fran Warren, Teacher's aide, Jericho Hill School for the Deaf (Vancouver). *Experience:* 13-year-old daughter and 19-year-old son, both prelingually deaf; latter attends Gallaudet College.

G. David Zink, M.A., Director, Division of Speech and Hearing, Ministry of Health, Province of British Columbia (Victoria). *Training:* audiology, speech pathology, education of the deaf. *Experience:* teacher of the deaf; clinical audiologist; research and development in prosthetic devices and provision of clinical services.

Staff of Hearing Disorders Program, Children's Hospital Diagnostic Centre, C. Dunella MacLean, M.D., C.M. (pediatrician and director); George Muller, M.A. (head, audiology and speech department, Children's Hospital); Kamal Deshpande, M.A. (audiologist and speech pathologist); Joan Pinkus, Ph.D. (psychologist); Jo Sleigh, M.S.W., and Pat Leibik, M.S.W. (social workers); and Barbara Shuman (teacher of the deaf).

UNITED STATES

Richard G. Brill, Ed.D., Retired Superintendent, California School for the Deaf (Riverside). *Training:* education of the deaf. *Experience:* several books on education of deaf children.

Frank Caccamise, Ph.D., Research Associate, Division of Communication Programs, National Technical Institute for the Deaf (Rochester,

N.Y.). *Training:* audiology. *Experience:* research on identification of visual impairment; technical signs used in academic/career settings; Total Communication programs for children and their families.

Ann Champ-Wilson, Co-Founder and Executive Director, Deafpride, Inc. (Washington, D.C.); formerly Treasurer, International Association of Parents of the Deaf. *Experience:* 15-year-old prelingually deaf son.

Bonnie Fairchild, President, International Association of Parents of the Deaf (Silver Spring, Maryland). *Experience:* 17-year-old prelingually deaf daughter.

Mervin D. Garretson, M.A., Special Assistant to the President, Gallaudet College (Washington, D.C.). *Training:* English; education of the deaf. *Experience:* deaf since age 5; wife severely hard-of-hearing; attended state residential school for 11 years; formerly Principal, Montana School for the Deaf, and Model Secondary School for the Deaf (Washington, D.C.); immediate Past President, National Association of the Deaf; International President, Commission on Pedagogy, World Federation of the Deaf.

Joanne Greenberg, Author of *In This Sign* and *I Never Promised You a Rose Garden* and other novels (Golden, Colorado). Honorary Doctor of Letters degrees from Gallaudet College and Western Maryland College. *Experience:* development of mental health services and first-aid training for deaf persons.

Mark T. Greenberg, Ph.D., Assistant Professor of Psychology, University of Washington (Seattle). *Training:* developmental and pediatric psychology. *Experience:* Advisory Board Member, Center on Deafness, University of California, San Francisco; research on early social communication and the effects of early intervention with deaf children.

Robert I. Harris, Ph.D., Clinical Psychologist and Coordinator, Child and Family Studies, St. Paul-Ramsey Medical Center's Mental Health and Hearing-Impaired Program; Assistant Professor of Psychiatry, University of Minnesota. *Training:* clinical psychology. *Experience:* prelingually deaf, married to a deaf woman.

Leo Jacobs, M.A., Retired educator and Coordinator of Continuing and Community Education, California School for the Deaf, Berkeley, California. *Experience:* prelingually deaf; deaf parents, wife, brother, child; residence counselor; Past President, Gallaudet College Alumni Association; first holder of Powrie Vaux Doctor Chair of Deaf Studies (1972–73) at Gallaudet College.

Barbara M. Kannapell, M.A., Co-Founder and President, Deafpride, Inc.; Linguistics Specialist, Gallaudet College (Washington, D.C.). *Training:* sociolinguistics. *Experience:* prelingually deaf, from a deaf family; Ph.D. candidate in sociolinguistics, Georgetown University; advocate of bilingual education for deaf children.

Robert K. Lennan, M.A., M.Ed., Ed.D., Superintendent, California School for the Deaf (Riverside). *Training:* physical education, history, education of the deaf, educational administration, educational psychology and instructional technology. *Experience:* dormitory counselor; physical education, elementary and secondary school teaching and administration; multiply handicapped deaf children.

Billie McDavitt, SEE-II Instructor, Wichita State University; Tutor-Interpreter, Wichita Public Schools (Wichita, Kansas). *Training:* English. *Experience:* 12-year-old son whose deafness began at age 5; Board Member, International Association of Parents of the Deaf.

Kathryn P. Meadow, Ph.D., Director, Child Development Research Unit, Research Institute, Gallaudet College; Executive Director, Kendall Demonstration Elementary School, (Washington, D.C.). *Training:* sociology. *Experience:* co-author of *Sound and Sign: Childhood Deafness and Mental Health* and of *Deafness and Child Development.*

Jacqueline Z. Mendelsohn, M.S., Executive Director, International Association of Parents of the Deaf (Silver Spring, Maryland). *Training:* psychology. *Experience:* 11-year-old prelingually deaf son, mainstreamed with an interpreter.

Donald F. Moores, Ph.D., Head, Teaching and Assessment Studies, Educational Research Laboratory, and Professor, Department of Educational Foundations and Research, Gallaudet College (Washington, D.C.). *Training:* psychology, psycholinguistics, education of the deaf. *Experience:* author of *Educating the Deaf* and of various research publications.

Jeffrey E. Nash, Ph.D., Associate Professor of Sociology and Linguistics, Macalester College (St. Paul, Minnesota). *Training:* sociology. *Experience:* 11-year-old prelingually deaf son; sociology of deafness and of sign language usage.

Lawrence Newman, M.A., Assistant Superintendent, California School for the Deaf (Riverside). *Training:* English, mathematics, administration. *Experience:* deaf from age 5, wife's parents are deaf, has 11-year-old prelingually deaf daughter; California Teacher of the Year, 1969.

Wilda W. Owens, Past President, International Association of Parents of the Deaf (1977–79). *Experience:* 31-year-old prelingually deaf son; charter member, Georgia Association of the Deaf Parent Chapter No. 4 and Georgia Registry of Interpreters for the Deaf.

Roslyn Rosen, M.A., Ed.D., Director, Special School of the Future Project, Gallaudet College (Washington, D.C.). *Training:* education of the deaf, communications, administration. *Experience:* prelingually deaf; deaf parents and sibling, mother of three prelingually deaf children; supervising teacher; vocational rehabilitation counselor; P.L. 94–142 coordinator.

Jerome D. Schein, Ph.D., Professor, Deafness Rehabilitation, and Director, Deafness Research and Training Center, New York University, New York. *Training:* clinical psychology. *Experience:* research, administration, deaf culture.

John G. Schroedel, Ph.D., Research Specialist, Educational Research Laboratory, Model Secondary School for the Deaf, Gallaudet College (Washington, D.C.). *Training:* sociology. *Experience:* prelingually deaf; research on attitudes toward, and social development of, people who are deaf.

Thomas and Louise Spradley. Louise is aide/tutor/interpreter for a junior high school mainstreaming program; Tom is co-author with his brother of *Deaf Like Me* (Sacramento, California). *Experience:* prelingually deaf 15-year-old daughter.

William C. Stokoe, Ph.D., Director, Linguistics Research Laboratory, Gallaudet College (Washington, D.C.); Visiting Fellow, Clare Hall, Cambridge University (England). *Training:* anthropology. *Experience:* originator of modern ASL research.

Roberta Thomas, M.A., Co-chairman, Philadelphia Area IAPD Action Alliance. *Training:* French and English. *Experience:* 4-year-old prelingually deaf son; advocacy for deaf children and their parents.

McCay Vernon, Ph.D., Professor of Psychology, Western Maryland College (Westminster); Powrie Vaux Doctor Chair of Deaf Studies, Gallaudet College, 1979–80; Editor, American Annals of the Deaf. *Training:* psychology. *Experience:* wife is deaf; research and advocacy on all aspects of hearing impairment; co-author of *They Grow in Silence*; expert on Usher's Syndrome.

UNITED KINGDOM

Mary Brennan, Lecturer in English and Linguistics, Principal Investigator, British Sign Language Research Project, Moray House College of Education, Edinburgh. *Training:* linguistics.

R. Conrad, Ph.D., Medical Research Council Applied Psychology Unit (Cambridge University). *Training:* psychology. *Experience:* author of *The Deaf Schoolchild* and basic research on cognitive processes in deaf children.

Clive Davis, C.Q.S.W., Dip. Deaf Welfare, Social Worker, Employment Services Officer, Royal National Institute for the Deaf (London). *Training:* social work. *Experience:* deaf from age 7; has 11-year-old prelingually deaf son; wife is prelingually deaf; involved in further education for deaf people and lectures to professionals about deafness.

John C. Denmark, M.B., Ch.B., D.P.M., F.R.C.Psych., Consultant Psychiatrist, Department of Psychiatry for the Deaf, Whittingham Hospital (Preston, Lancashire). *Training:* medicine (psychiatry). *Experience:* son of headmaster, Liverpool School for the Deaf; brother was headmaster of School for the Deaf in Belfast, Northern Ireland.

Lionel Evans, M.A., M.Sc., Ph.D., Headmaster, Northern Counties School for the Deaf (Newcastle-Upon-Tyne); Hon. Lecturer in Education, University of Newcastle-Upon-Tyne. Powrie Vaux Doctor Chair of Deaf Studies, Gallaudet College, 1980–1981. *Training:* education, psychology, audiology. *Experience:* active in re-introducing Total Communication methods to the U.K.

Margaret M. Keir, M.A., Head Teacher, Garvel Deaf Centre (Greenock, Scotland). *Training:* education. *Experience:* introduced Total Communication; developing application of BSL Research Project.

Paddy Ladd, M.A., Co-founder and formerly General Secretary, National Union of the Deaf (London). *Training:* social work, youth work. *Experience:* postlingually deaf; English literature, linguistics, modern cultural studies; produced first deaf-run TV program in the U.K., 1979.

Maureen MacKenzie, Social Psychologist, Donaldson's School for the Deaf (Edinburgh). *Training:* psychology, counseling with deaf people, sign languages. *Experience:* research on sign language in educational settings and social factors in integration.

George Montgomery, Ph.D., Psychologist, Donaldson's School for the Deaf (Edinburgh). *Training:* psychology. *Experience:* research on language in deaf children; mental health and deafness.

AUSTRALIA

Raymond Jeanes, B.A., B.Ed., Lecturer, Institute of Special Education, Burwood State College (Melbourne). *Training:* education of the deaf. *Experience:* research on Australian Sign Language.

Desmond Power, Ph.D., Director, Centre for Human Development Studies, Mt. Gravatt College of Advanced Education (Mt. Gravatt, Queensland). *Training:* psychology and education of the deaf. *Experience:* research on language development and on multiply handicapped deaf children; training of teachers of the deaf; now developing early intervention program.

Brian E. Reynolds, Principal, Victorian School for Deaf Children (Melbourne, Victoria). *Training:* education and education of the deaf (Licentiate, Australian Association of Teachers of the Deaf). *Experience:* paternal grandparents were deaf and attended Victorian School; father was superintendent of Victorian Adult Deaf Society for over 30 years.

DENMARK

Lars von der Lieth, M.A., Associate Professor of Psychology, University of Copenhagen. *Training:* developmental and clinical psychology. *Experience:* International Chairman, Psychological Commis-

sion, World Federation of the Deaf; organizer, Group for the Mental Health of the Deaf.

FRANCE

Danielle Bouvet, Linguist and speech pathologist/therapist for profoundly deaf children, Fondation Borel-Maisonny (Paris); Professeur de Psychopedagogie de la Langue Maternelle, University of Geneva (Switzerland). *Training:* speech, linguistics, psychology. *Experience:* introduced bilingual education for deaf preschoolers, sign language classes for parents, TV programs in sign language.

ISRAEL

Jerry Reichstein, M.A., Ed.D., Coordinator, Hearing Impairment Program, School of Education, Tel Aviv University; Professional Consultant, Shema Centres. *Training:* special education, education of the deaf, audiology. *Experience:* hard-of-hearing (60 dB level) from one year of age; educational rehabilitation of the hearing-impaired of all ages.

MALAYSIA

Tan Chin Guan, Chairman, Society for the Deaf in Selangor and the Federal Territory, 1978–79. *Training:* education. *Experience:* he and his wife (virologist Dr. Dora Tan) helped with the promotion of Total Communication in Malaysia; vice-chairman of Ministry of Education subcommittee to implement Total Communication.

SWEDEN

Brita Bergman, Fil.Mag., Researcher and Project Leader, Department of Linguistics, University of Stockholm. *Training:* linguistics. *Experience:* expert on Signed Swedish; lecturer on linguistics and sign language; directs research project on Swedish Sign Language.

Kerstin Nordén, Ph.D., Assistant Professor of Educational Psychology, Malmö School of Education, Lund University (Malmö). *Training:* psychology. *Experience:* has 34-year-old prelingually deaf son; member of board of directors, School for the Deaf, Lund.

CAN'T YOUR CHILD HEAR?
A Guide for
Those Who Care about
Deaf Children

Chapter 1

DEAFNESS
A Difference to be Accepted, or a Defect to be Corrected?

You have every right to feel disappointment, resentment, and guilt. You have suffered a loss. Your dreams have been shattered. But as you begin to learn what it is like to be deaf, and how to communicate with your deaf boy or girl, we believe you will recapture the dreams you had for your new baby. [T. Spradley, personal communication, 1980]

INTRODUCTION

The fundamental fact about children who are deaf is that they communicate in a different way. Their parents, 90% of whom have normal hearing, find that there is a break in the natural pattern of communication, and that they must somehow learn to cope with this difference.

In this first chapter, we examine why the question in the chapter title is significant. We also set out a few of the goals we believe to be important for deaf children, for their families, and for those who work with them.

Deaf children are not all the same; there are several important factors that can influence how their deafness affects them. This makes it difficult to write a book that applies equally to *all* children who are deaf. We discuss in the preface whom the book is intended for and the extent to which it is relevant for different kinds and degrees of

1

deafness. If you have not already read the preface, we strongly suggest that you do so now.

CONTROVERSIES AND CONFUSION

Of all the areas of childhood disability, deafness is likely to be the most confusing and controversial. This is probably because the ability to speak is so closely connected in our minds with thinking, communicating, and intelligence. At least for those children whose hearing loss begins in very early life, the lack of hearing is not their most serious problem—instead, it is their difficulty in developing an adequate communication system.

Parents are sometimes given conflicting or confusing advice concerning their deaf child. They are told to "treat him as normal," while getting constant indications from relatives, friends, the general public, and their own observations that the child is, in many ways, very different from what is usually thought of as normal. In addition, parents too often share the public's misconception that science will soon have an answer to all problems. Some parents and professionals may be more impressed with electronic hardware than with the knowledge and experience of people who are deaf.

For 200 years the major controversy in the field of deafness has been what method(s) of communication (oral, manual) should be used with the deaf child. The different approaches to communication can profoundly affect almost every area of family life: hopes and expectations; selection of educational and recreational programs; whether friends should be hearing, deaf, or both; and how best to include the deaf child in family communication. Although some professional readers may be tired of hearing about "the controversy," it cannot be avoided.

A very brief and necessarily oversimplified look at some of the differences in points of view of those who do and

Table 1. Some Controversies in Views of Deafness

Area of Concern	Auditory/Oral Group	Total Communication Group
View of deaf people	A handicapped group	A linguistic minority
Model for success	The hearing child or adult	The successful deaf person
Natural language of a deaf child	Language of the hearing majority	Visual sign language or sign system
View of sign languages	Often seen as defective, primitive, even repulsive; should be avoided	Valued as clear, complete, expressive, beautiful, and legitimate languages
Acceptable ways of communicating	Amplified speech plus speechreading and speech training	Same, including signing, mime, fingerspelling, and body language
Effects of signing on speech	Usually claim it impairs development	No negative effects, or may even improve it
Educational role of deaf adults	None if not oral	Important as teachers, role models, counselors, and administrators
Association with other deaf people	No benefits; avoid those who sign	Necessary for a normal life
Total integration into hearing society	A realistic and desirable goal	A difficult or impossible goal for most; partial integration is encouraged, but extent is variable

those who do not advocate the use of sign language is presented in Table 1.

IMPORTANCE OF PARENTS

Despite controversies over methods of communication, there is one area of complete agreement: parents are essential for the deaf child's emotional, social, and linguistic development. All the professionals in the world cannot provide a substitute for them. We all assume that parents should gain some satisfaction from the demanding tasks of child-rearing. However, this may not be easy to sustain when conflicting advice creates uncertainty and lack of confidence, and when life as a parent seems to consist of wondering whether you are doing the right thing, and of believing that, if you aren't, you will bear the eventual responsibility.

Some parents find at least temporary relief by clinging exclusively to one approach or to one expert's advice, as if they feel that all the answers are already available. This is an understandable reaction, probably reinforced by previous experiences with physicians, who treat curable or minor illnesses with great success. Unfortunately, deafness cannot be treated in this way; it requires a much greater maturity of knowledge and attitudes. Most hearing people, including some professionals, have little but ignorance to depend upon in their approach to deafness.

CONFUSION CAN'T BE AVOIDED

We have written this book with the belief that, in the long run, it is better for parents to make their own decisions after considering the facts, the different interpretations of those facts, and the opposing value systems derived from them. This often results in some confusion and suffering before a reasonable comfort level is reached. Although you might wish to avoid this painful process, it is part of the adjustment to any major life change, and with increasing interest in and publicity about deafness, it is almost impossible to insulate yourself from the controversies about deafness and from the ultimate need to make decisions about it.

Another confusing element that should be understood is that in some respects the uncertainty about rearing a deaf child is only a little different from the uncertainty about raising any child when the old dependable prescriptions of what is "right" and "wrong" have withered away. Should physical punishment be used? At what point should limits be set? Is it good or bad for parents to exclude a child from parental activities? Should children of different ages have different bedtimes? How much should children share family problems? Little scientific evidence is available to answer these questions or others like them as they apply to any family; we doubt there ever will be. As de Bono (1979) has stated: "Decision is the application of values to action" (p. 23); "No decision is perfect. Most decisions have to be based on inadequate knowledge and some guesswork" (p. 176).

Although we certainly don't want to imply that every part of daily life with a deaf child is complicated, it is nevertheless true that having a child who is different creates new situations and feelings requiring different coping skills. Few (if any) parents are likely to have this special knowledge when their child's disability is identified, because only about one child in a thousand is deaf.

THE REALITY OF DEAFNESS

In the past it was rare for deaf children or their parents to encounter deaf adults at all, much less as equals. It may not be surprising, then, that some deaf children believed that there simply were no deaf adults and that they would eventually turn into "hearing people." Similarly, some parents hoped that, through the use of hearing aids and diligent speech training, their child would blend into the larger hearing world, and that many or most of the characteristics that identified their child as deaf would disappear. We believe that, for most severely and profoundly deaf children, this is a false and indeed dangerous expectation—dangerous because persistent false hope delays the process of parents' accepting their child's deafness.

What is this process of "acceptance?" We all wish to be proud of our children. The identification of our child as "different" or "handicapped" threatens this budding pride,

and we need ways to restore it. If we have no way of learning
that deaf adults can have a full and satisfying life (although
it may be different from ours in some ways), what path is
open to restore that pride? Perhaps only the dream of
"overcoming" or "bypassing" deafness remains. Here all our
fears, prejudices, and stereotypes about deaf people come
into play. Think of the many negative expressions we
encounter as we are growing up: "falling on deaf ears,"
meaning unresponsive; "deaf and dumb," suggesting stupid;
"deaf-mute," implying an inability to express oneself; and so
on. It is only when you can correct your perceptions of
persons who are deaf and can find a sense of shared
humanity that your horizons may be broadened to include
the real possibility of pride in the deaf child—with or without
speech. It is this fundamental process that we wish to start,
or to facilitate, by means of this book. This is why we have
chosen to follow this chapter not with the traditional details
of diagnosis or with the application of hearing aids, but with
a presentation of what it is like to be deaf (Chapter 2). In
doing so we are not, by any means, downgrading the
usefulness of speech for those who can acquire it, nor the
great importance of learning to use the language of the
surrounding majority of hearing people. Dignity and appreciation, however, are more basic psychologically and are
indeed crucial to the realization of these educational
accomplishments.

In the next part, we discuss our focus and our definition
of deafness.

OUR FOCUS

We do not mean to suggest that "success" will automatically
follow from an application of the concepts presented here.
In fact, we are encouraging you, the reader, to explore and
to re-define the values you may feel are included in the idea
of "success." This is easier to do if you understand the
different ways, now and in the past, of approaching the

rearing and education of deaf children. Our own point of view favors what is called "Total Communication." (Total Communication is defined and fully discussed in Chapter 12, but for our purposes here it includes the use of all means of communication useful to the child and family, including sign language.) Our goal will be reached if those who care for deaf children will constructively use both the controversies over deafness and their own confusion about it by thinking, asking questions, discussing, and thinking again. Their eventual decisions may be different because no one set of methods suits all deaf children or all families.

DEFINITION OF DEAFNESS

The use of the word "deaf" is often confusing and inconsistent. Whom do we mean when we refer to "deaf children?" Some experts (and some deaf people) deplore the use of this word, arguing that hardly anyone is really deaf, because there is usually some residual hearing left. They feel that referring to someone as "deaf" may be a self-fulfilling prophecy, because parents and others may give up on the intensive training of residual hearing through amplification. The term "hearing-impaired" has come to refer to all degrees of hearing loss, and some books on the subject never use the word "deaf." However, because the word "deaf" is firmly entrenched in popular usage, and need not imply there is no hearing at all, we will use it in accordance with the following definitions:

> A *deaf person* is one whose hearing is disabled to an extent . . . that precludes the understanding of speech through the ear alone, without or with the use of a hearing aid. A *hard-of-hearing person* is one whose hearing is disabled to an extent . . . that makes difficult, but does not preclude, the understanding of speech through the ear alone, without or with a hearing aid. [Moores, 1978b, p. 5]

Moores also gives useful brief definitions of two other terms that will be encountered throughout this book:

> *Prelingual deafness* refers to the condition of persons whose deafness was present at birth or occurred at an age prior to the development of speech and language. *Postlingual deafness* refers to the condition of persons whose deafness

occurred at an age following the spontaneous acquisition of speech and language.
[p. 7]

There are two other terms that can be confusing.
Congenital refers to deafness present at birth, whatever the
cause. *Hereditary* or *genetic* deafness usually is congenital, but
sometimes its effects only become apparent later in life.

There are some children who function as "deaf" (although their hearing losses are not very severe) because of
other disabilities. They may, for example, hear some speech
sounds but be unable to attach meaning to them. A few very
deaf people are able to function as hard-of-hearing persons.
The ability to make use of amplification will vary from one
situation to another. Many hard-of-hearing persons are
"socially deaf" when in a group or where there is considerable
noise.

Another consideration is how people define *themselves*.
For example, some profoundly deaf persons might prefer
the label "hearing-impaired" or "hard-of-hearing" because
they were taught to avoid referring to themselves as "deaf"
and were discouraged from associating with deaf people.
Some hard-of-hearing people choose to associate primarily
with deaf persons and label themselves "deaf." These are
just a few of the complications attached to labeling.

We will use the term "hearing-impaired" only to refer to
both deaf and hard-of-hearing individuals.

DESIRABLE GOALS

Goals for Deaf Children

To grow up as fully participating members of their families,
    with the same basic opportunities as any child, and with the
    firmest possible sense of self-worth, dignity, and acceptance
    (regardless of how clearly they speak)
To acquire a useful knowledge of English (including the spoken
    form, to the extent possible) and the social skills necessary
    to interact with hearing people (bilingualism)
To have relatives and self-selected friends with whom they can
    communicate easily

To develop a rich early-language base, not only to form warm
  relationships with other people, but also to express wonder,
  curiosity, love, disappointment, anger, and fear; to ask
  questions and receive answers about natural occurrences in
  everyday life
To have respect for other people, their language, ways of life,
  and accomplishments, including hearing-impaired persons
  (biculturalism)
To gain reasonable tolerance for the ignorance of most hearing
  people about deafness

Goals for Families of Deaf Children

Knowledge of basic facts about deafness
Awareness and understanding of their own feelings (including
  negative ones about deafness and their deaf child)
Sharing of experiences and feelings with other parents, to know
  that they are not alone
Pride in their deaf child as a person (without demanding
  intelligible speech as a prerequisite)
A communication medium (signing) that is clear and that can be
  used during the deaf child's earliest years, so that all
  experiences are available for learning
Support (when needed) by compassionate professionals who
  know the limitations of their own knowledge
A sense of proportion that takes into account not only the needs
  of the child who is deaf, but also those of other family
  members
A willingness to let the deaf child develop independence,
  including taking reasonable risks and making decisions and
  mistakes
Joy in seeing a precious family member develop with a
  minimum of frustration
A sense of humor to carry them through life's darker moments
Enough energy to be advocates and even activists when
  necessary

Goals for Professionals

Ability to take parental concerns seriously
Acceptance of deaf people as equals, with a focus on strengths
  as well as limitations

Caution in applying their experience with other disabilities to
    deaf persons
Awareness of major trends in the field, or willingness to learn
    about them
Openness to new ideas
Compassion

CONCLUSIONS

Deafness is a fact of life. People who are deaf lead lives that
are in some ways different, but not inferior to the lives of
people with normal hearing. If you can accept deafness as
a difference, not a defect, you will find that it will help you
to find joy and delight in raising a "normal" child. Some of
these delights are the same as those experienced with a
hearing child, some are different—but they are just as
fulfilling. The chapters that follow explore how this insight
fits with all the other things that parents can do.

Good general references for parents who are not yet
very experienced with deafness are: Furth (1973), Mindel
and Vernon (1971), Naiman and Schein (1978), and Pahz
and Pahz (1977).

SUMMARY

1. Deaf children need to communicate in a different way; this poses special problems for their parents, 90% of whom have normal hearing.

2. This book is intended for parents and professional workers. It is most applicable to those deaf children who cannot acquire language through hearing, even with amplification (severe and profound deafness with prelingual onset).

3. The most serious obstacle deaf children face is not the lack of hearing, but their difficulty in developing an adequate communication system.

4. Deafness is probably the most controversial and confusing of childhood disabilities.

5. The so-called oral-manual controversy is the most deep-rooted and enduring of the disputes and can affect many areas of living for families with deaf members.

6. Because only about one child in a thousand is deaf, few hearing parents have any prior knowledge of how to raise a deaf child; yet everyone agrees that the parents' role is essential.

7. The uncertainty of raising a deaf child is, in some ways, only an exaggeration of the normal uncertainties of rearing any child.

8. Denial of the differences that deafness imposes can cause serious problems. This can occur when parents try to restore their pride in their child. Pride should not be based upon the extent to which their child can bypass deafness, but on the finding of shared and valued qualities, regardless of deafness.

9. Definitions of "success" need to be re-examined.

10. Some desirable goals for deaf children, families, and professionals are presented in capsule form, to be elaborated later. These are based on the

idea that deaf children should grow up with
their inevitable differences accepted, by
themselves and by those who care about them.
These differences should not prevent a fulfilling
life for child or family.

Chapter 2

WHAT IS IT LIKE TO BE DEAF?

It's very difficult to know what it's like being deaf if you've never been deaf.
. . . I worry if she'll get married. I mean they do get married, don't they? . . . She
won't be able to hear anybody tell her they love her and things like that. [Quotes
from three English mothers, taken from Gregory, 1976, pp. 210–211]

In an age when communication is so important, not to understand what is going
on around you is a very frightening experience. You withdraw from things and
stay by yourself. Or you try to find others who are like yourself so you can share
experiences. [Lattin, 1975, p. 19]

NECESSITY FOR AN OVERALL PERSPECTIVE

Without some realistic and expanding knowledge of the lives
of deaf people, you as parent of a deaf child are at the mercy
of your ignorance, like the three mothers quoted above. We
believe it is absolutely essential to acquire at least a beginning
awareness of how deaf people live before proceeding to any
other aspects of deafness.

The title of this chapter poses a challenging question.
Whenever the question is asked, "What is it like to be deaf?"
it is important to be clear about who is answering. Is it a
hearing or a deaf parent? A teacher of the deaf? An
audiologist? A physician? A relative of a deaf child? A deaf
adult with or without much formal education? Depending
upon each person's background and knowledge, the answer
is likely to be different. Many descriptions and images of
what it is like to be deaf are available to us (Batson and
Bergman, 1976; Bowe and Sternberg, 1973; Braddock and
Crammatte, 1975; Deafpride, 1976; Greenberg, 1970; Higgins, 1980; and Watson, 1973).

Human beings are selective; they do not see all of reality, rather they automatically construct it based upon their individual experiences and expectations (Wegner and Vallacher, 1977). As a parent, you will have fewer problems about whom to believe if you realize that different perspectives, opinions, and descriptions are only natural. When you recognize the diversity of deaf people and of those working with them, you will be more fully aware of the total picture. There is, however, always more to learn. No one person, deaf or hearing, layman or professional, can convey a description of *all* deaf people.

THE HEARING PERSON'S BIAS

Hearing persons are handicapped when they try to understand deaf people. They have lived for their entire lives using and depending upon their hearing and speech. Just as sighted people have tremendous difficulties imagining what it would be like for a blind person to dream without vision, so life without hearing and intelligible speech is probably impossible to imagine except as the loss of something of great value.

It is perhaps this powerful fact that gives deafness a negative meaning for most hearing persons. Except for the relatively few deaf children whose hearing loss occurred after language developed (the postlingually deaf), there is no reason to believe that all deaf children feel a sense of personal loss until they compare themselves to hearing children and encounter the attitudes of society toward deafness. Their awareness of a difference and their regret over some things they cannot do are *not* the same as the grief of a hearing individual over a lost body function.

THE DEAF COMMUNITY

If someone were to ask you, a hearing reader of this book, what it is like to live in the hearing world, the question might seem unfair, vague, or impossible to answer. You know that there is no single "hearing world." Perhaps you could make some general statements, but could not truly describe the life experience and inner feelings of hearing persons—at least not *all* hearing persons.

Neither is it a simple question for people who are deaf to describe a "deaf world." Contrary to anything you may be told, there is no single "deaf world" or "deaf community." Deaf persons relate to each other and to hearing people in many different ways.

Other factors may partially determine how deaf people function socially: when they became deaf, whether they had the benefits of good, early two-way communication in their homes, their degree of useful hearing, their school opportunities, their native intelligence, and their individual personalities.

Despite these warnings about generalizing, we do want to present a few important facts about deaf people as a group, without any assumption that all of these will apply equally to all individuals. The following findings are derived from two American studies (Schein, 1968; Schein and Delk, 1974) and from Scandinavian experience (von der Lieth, 1978).

1. About 10% of deaf children have deaf parents.
2. Of the 60% of deaf adults who marry, 85%–95% marry other deaf persons. Such marriages are more stable than those that are mixed (hearing and deaf). Overall divorce rates are comparable to those in the hearing population. Of the offspring of deaf couples, only 10%–12% are themselves deaf.
3. In families where the parents are deaf, over 90% communicate with each other and their children primarily in sign language, although speech is also used simultaneously by many of those with adequate skills.
4. Only a minority of hearing parents use sign language with their deaf children, and few of these do so from the time of diagnosis. This situation is changing now in North America.
5. Two-thirds of deaf persons are members of at least one organization of deaf people; half of these are members of two or more (von der Lieth, 1978).

6. Educationally, the majority of deaf high school graduates
   are far behind their hearing peers; their average reading
   level is comparable to that of a 9–10-year-old hearing child,
   in spite of average intelligence. Although most deaf adults
   are self-supporting, their average annual earnings are lower
   than those of comparable hearing individuals.
7. In some developed countries, groups of deaf people have
   established their own cultural societies, theater, publications,
   television programs, athletic organizations (including World
   Games of the Deaf), clubs and conventions, businesses,
   beauty pageants, and leadership training programs. (See
   Chapter 14.)

Leo Jacobs, a born-deaf teacher of mathematics, has
written an excellent book, entitled *A Deaf Adult Speaks Out*,
that should be read by all parents. Jacobs's deaf family
members include his parents, his wife, and one of his two
children. In addition to receiving a Master's degree, in
1972–73 he was honored as the first holder of the Powrie
Doctor Chair of Deaf Studies at Gallaudet College in Washington, D.C., the world's only liberal arts college primarily
for hearing-impaired students. Jacobs's views and experiences, especially as they relate to minority-group dynamics
(see also Vernon and Makowsky, 1969) follow:

> I never noticed my own handicap nor came up against discrimination or unfair
> treatment until I began my own personal contacts with hearing people when I
> entered school . . . I felt more handicapped from the treatment I received at the
> hands of hearing people than from my deafness . . . The real ills of deaf people
> lie more with minority group dynamics than with their deafness [p. 99]. . . . they
> are subject to the same problems that other minority groups face: the demand
> that the minority people come up to the expectations of the majority, and the
> majority's utter disregard for the real needs of the minority group; and in addition
> the preconceived opinions, the prejudices, the power structure, the self-
> perpetuation, the superiority complex (paternalism), and the authority held by the
> members of the majority over the minority segment. The majority also has the
> melting pot, or manifest destiny concept of minority group persons—that all of
> them have to be the same [p. 61]. . . . No matter how large a deaf population
> may be in any given area, it is still only a very small fraction of the general
> population, and therefore maintains the warm, close-knit, and folksy atmosphere
> of a small town or village where everyone is acquainted with everybody else.
> [Jacobs, 1974, p. 71]

This description should not be taken to mean that deaf
people have no antagonisms to subgroups within their

own community, or that as a group they are more tolerant and less prejudiced than the larger society of which they are a part.

DIFFERENCE OR DEFECT?

Chapter 1 introduced the idea of interpreting the problems, challenges, and tasks of rearing a deaf child either as a developmental difference to be accepted or as a defect to be corrected. We can illustrate the two approaches by making some comparisons between the deaf children of deaf parents and those of hearing parents.

Deaf parents typically accept their deaf baby as a normal child, who will be like them in most respects, and therefore they see very few problems. They know what to expect and are acquainted with other deaf parents who have successfully raised deaf children. From the start, they communicate easily with their child and have an overall attitude that is probably no different from a hearing parent of a hearing child.

The situation in hearing families is usually quite different. There is a high risk that their deaf children will be reminded daily, year after year, that they are different and that their speech is not right. Even though this is done with the best of intentions, it may make it difficult to achieve a close bond between parents and child. Parents should communicate, not evaluate communication.

No other "handicap" has anything similar to the 200-year-long controversy over which form of communication a deaf child should use. Because most deaf adults whom you will meet have had hearing parents, the professional advice given them is usually to avoid sign language. Therefore, they have been denied a clear system of two-way communication within their own families.

Attitudes toward sign language have had a major impact on deaf people, and they have been put in an extraordinary position because the great majority use sign language as adults, regardless of their education. It is used in clubs,

conferences, and educational programs after school is finished, yet their language is not shared by their families or
by their teachers, and it has not been given a place of dignity
by those who help mold their self-concept.

The opinions that follow are the negative attitudes of
two leading oralists. The first is Father van Uden of the
Netherlands, who feels that sign language is not only defective, but keeps its users at a subhuman level:

> It is said, that signing is the way of communication most natural to the deaf. This
> is true in the sense that—without help—they will never reach higher commu-
> nicative codes than signs and some attempts at lipreading and speaking. So
> crawling over the floor will be the way of locomotion most natural to handicapped
> persons with only two short stumps for legs . . . But now we can fit them with
> prostheses, by means of which they can learn to walk in a more human way, up
> to the same level as their fellow-men. This way of locomotion will be more natural
> to them as *human beings*. In the same sense, by good education, we can develop
> the attempts at lipreading and speaking of the deaf up to oral conversation, to
> oral language, by means of which the deaf can live with their hearing fellow-
> men in a more human way. And this oral language appears to be more natural
> to them *as human beings*. [van Uden, 1968, p. 75]

In a preface to van Uden's book, the late Sir Alexander
Ewing, one of the great advocates of pure oralism, stated:

> The Reverend van Uden has subjected use of signs and finger-spelling . . . to
> psycholinguistic analysis. He concludes that their disadvantages are very grave
> and that there should be no place for them. [p. 5]

Father van Uden (1974) also stated that the use of sign
language creates "a gigantic problem . . . with regard to
religious instruction (p. 236) . . . A pictorial way of thinking
. . . impedes an ascent to selfless love and authentic Christi-
anity" (p. 238).

The attitudes represented by these quotations may be
considered extreme; no doubt some oralists who are familiar
with modern research on sign languages would not endorse
them. Nevertheless, van Uden, who still travels around the
world as an honored expert, has not changed his views in
the past 12 years, and these dramatic quotations should serve
to alert us to similar but less clearly expressed opinions that
quite commonly affect deaf people.

After the Norman (French) conquest of Britain in 1066,
the ruling classes felt that English was a defective language,

not suitable for use at court or in polite society. This attitude may seem hard to believe now that English is a major world language. Similar attitudes have held sway over other languages or dialects. [A good general description of what has been called "linguistic chauvinism" can be found in Farb (1974).] We now know from linguistic studies that all naturally evolved languages have equal potential, and that negative attitudes toward sign languages are no more justified than the prejudice against English mentioned above.

CONTACT OF DEAF PERSONS WITH HEARING PERSONS

Encounters of minority groups with the larger society surrounding them often produce a well-developed sense of humor. Deaf persons are no exception—an entire book (Holcomb, 1977) has been devoted to the subject. Here we present a brief excerpt from another work:

> There is that inevitable time when you get a chest x-ray. The technician says, "Take a deep breath and hold it." Then he disappears for ages while you slowly turn purple waiting for him to come back so you'll know it is over. And how about the eye examination—how can you possibly lip-read with those drops in your eyes? Or the proctoscopic examination . . . how, in heaven's name, is the deaf patient expected to communicate in the dark in THAT position? [Jordan, 1971, p. 14]

Such misunderstandings are common between *any* two groups with different ways or needs. Deaf people who learn to manage well in these situations have more than a good sense of humor; they also have developed skills and strategies useful for getting through these predicaments and for helping hearing persons feel more comfortable with them (Higgins, 1980). You and your deaf child can learn a great deal from them. Sometimes, however, not all deaf individuals will be helpful. Some contacts may be less than a pleasure, but something can be learned from this, too.

By and large, deaf people think visually and are very observant. If you can learn to do this yourself, it will be easier to understand the world as seen by your deaf child.

Sooner or later you will probably be alone with several deaf people without the skills to communicate well with them; or you may be with another hearing person in a group of deaf people and feel a strong urge to communicate with the hearing person and not with the deaf people. These situations may help you to understand better what it is that deaf people experience in a reversed set of circumstances.

One of our parent resource people eloquently expressed her awareness of the potential contribution of deaf adults: "I cannot adequately express the gratitude I personally feel for the caring and sensitivity of the deaf adults who helped me *understand*, and therefore enriched my son's future immeasurably."

RESPONSIBILITY AND COMMUNICATION

Deaf people are often characterized as "immature." This means, in part, that on the average they have less general information, that their goals tend to be short- rather than long-range, and, that they may be less likely than hearing persons to think through the consequences of their actions.

Although these impressions may not be surprising, there seems to be little reason to believe that immaturity is inevitable; the lack of early communication within the family is cause enough for restricted growth because it deprives deaf children of the learning opportunities that are taken for granted with hearing children. This "immaturity" is largely, if not completely, preventable.

It is also important for deaf children to be given responsibility. A comparison study of 120 deaf children and their families with the same number of hearing children and their families was made in the Greater Vancouver area (Freeman, Malkin, and Hastings, 1975). Parents were asked to check off the independent activities they would permit their child to engage in. Deaf children were allowed to do less than hearing children of the same age. It seems that to be deaf with hearing parents may mean that you will be overprotected and denied an important area of development.

Sometimes the fact that deaf children can accept responsibility is not understood. Testimony in the British House of Commons by a Member of Parliament (Michael Morris) who was seeking special benefits for some of his constituents with deaf children included the following remarkable statements, which were not questioned:

> . . . whenever any of the children want to go out to take part in society, as we would all want them to do, they have to be accompanied. There is no chance of any of them going alone. . . . Their lack of ability to communicate—they can do so only by sign language—injures their personalities. . . . They will naturally also have behaviour problems. . . . [Hansard, debate records of the British Parliament, March 19, 1976]

We would like to emphasize that this is *not* what it is like to be deaf!

Deaf adults often report that they missed much of what was said in a hearing family: *why* things happen, *why* you are allowed to do something at one time and not at another, and *why* people feel and react the way they do. Seeing that deaf persons can accept responsibility should help you to present your child with reasonable expectations and to see the need for early two-way communication that will enable you to give explanations when you are asked "why?" A Total Communication approach fosters inclusion of your deaf child in family activities.

CONCLUSIONS

Deaf persons are as different from one another as hearing persons. In spite of some special problems that they must overcome because they have a minority group status and because their parents usually do not share that same status, it is important for you to know that deaf people can be as happy and productive, or as sad and unproductive, as hearing people. Much depends upon their opportunities and relationships as they are growing up.

   Progress can always be looked at in two ways: how far
you have come, and how far you must still go. Much progress
has been made by people who are deaf, but a great deal of
work still needs to be done. The remainder of this book
attempts to make both points clear.

SUMMARY

1. Hearing people must make a special effort to dispel the stereotypes of deafness. Their own experiences, which they take for granted, tend to give them the wrong impression—that life as a deaf person involves a constant sense of personal loss.

2. Stereotypes can make it more difficult for you as a parent to have reasonable hopes and expectations for your own deaf child.

3. There is considerable variation within the group called "the deaf community," and there is no single "deaf world," just as there is no single "hearing world."

4. Deaf adults have much to offer to deaf children and to their hearing parents.

5. Many (but not all) of the problems deaf people face are not inherent in deafness itself, but are related to what has been called "minority group dynamics," or attitudes of hearing people toward deaf people. This includes the condemnation of sign languages as defective or primitive.

6. Deaf people have developed their own organizations and find them to be valuable.

7. Although in the past deaf children were often inadvertently disadvantaged in their own hearing families, this situation is slowly improving.

8. Finding that you can like deaf people, lose your fear of them, and not see them as anything less than human beings will help you to feel better about your child.

Chapter 3

SUSPICION, DELAY, AND DIAGNOSIS

Most mothers interviewed had thought that their child was deaf long before it was officially confirmed. . . . On the one side you have professionals emphasizing the importance of early diagnosis and early auditory training, and on the other, mothers feeling there is something wrong with their child and help not being forthcoming. . . . It is hard to admit one's child is deaf, and harder still to maintain this position against "the experts." [Gregory, 1976, pp. 148, 156–157]

THE PROBLEM

Several surveys have shown that the diagnosis of deafness, which is essential before a child can start a program, tends to be unnecessarily delayed (Freeman, et al., 1975; Wong and Shah, 1979). This may be difficult to understand in a world where new medical advances are taken for granted. Bad feelings toward those who seem responsible for the delay may create obstacles for future cooperation. In this chapter we examine some of reasons why a delayed diagnosis is common. Then we discuss parental reactions to the diagnosis and what can be done to reduce its impact.

PARENTAL OBSERVATIONS OF HEARING LOSS

Under ordinary conditions, those who live with the child are better able than any test to detect that something is wrong (Wong and Shah, 1979). You may not be sure that it is deafness, but when there is no expected response to loud noises (such as a vacuum cleaner or fire engine) and there is a failure of speech development, you are likely to conclude that something is wrong. Unfortunately, the sensitivity of deaf babies' vision and vibration sense may occasionally produce a response that looks normal to those testing the hearing (physician, parent, or relative).

Professionals have different levels of experience; some will be good and others poor at identifying childhood deafness and at parent counseling.

How soon congenital deafness is suspected depends upon the severity of the loss—the more hearing that is left (residual hearing), the later the suspicion. Although there is no consistent pattern within families, one frequently troublesome occurrence that was found was that the mother was alone in believing that something was wrong. This was reported by 38% of the families in our Vancouver-area survey (Freeman et al., 1975). In this case, the mother is isolated with her worry because she feels that no one agrees with her judgment. One of the English mothers interviewed by Gregory (1976, p. 100) stated: "I was just sheer relieved to know that it wasn't me going mad. . . . I thought that if it went on much longer at home and that child was supposed to be normal, I'd go off me rocker." When the mother is eventually proved correct, she may harbor resentment against those who failed to support her. Some mothers even have difficulty accepting reassurance later on, when they have other anxieties about their child. It is as if they are continuing to believe in the rightness of their own worries.

Physicians who treat parents as if there were no problem ("he'll grow out of it"), or as if the parents were to blame, should be more sensitive to parental desperation and anxiety and should refer them for another opinion. In this way, much future anger and bitterness could be avoided.

In the Vancouver study, deafness was first suspected by one or both parents in 75% of the cases, and by physicians only 5% of the time. The average age of suspicion was 10 months for profound losses and 16 months for severe deafness. [These findings are similar to those reported in the United States (see, for example, Fellendorf and Harrow, 1970).]

THE DELAY

If you suspect something is wrong with your child, you will probably report your concern to your family doctor, pediatrician, or public health nurse. What happens then? In the previously mentioned Vancouver study (Freeman et al., 1975), the delay in diagnosis from the time of suspicion was almost 9 months for profound deafness and almost 16 months for severe deafness. There are several aspects of deafness that help account for this delay. They are summarized by Schlesinger (1974, p. 22) as the "infrequency, invisibility, uniqueness, and the sharing of symptomatology with other childhood disorders." Most physicians never encounter a deaf baby; there is nothing impressive to "see." Some behavior, such as cooing, babbling, and responsiveness to loud noises and movement may be normal. There are also many factors that may account for the things that concern you and for your child's responses during the doctor's exam. (Behavior of a baby in the office may be very different from behavior in the home.) Finally, many physicians tend to overvalue their brief examination in comparison with the countless observations made by parents (Schlesinger, 1971).

An additional and often forgotten factor is that although your child's behavior and performance are all-important to you, the doctor is dealing with probabilities: how likely is it that your worry about deafness will prove to be correct? Reassurances that your child is normal will often be accurate, but those that are wrong may be long remembered! In the Vancouver study, one-half of family physicians consulted by parents of children later found to be deaf did not agree that the child was deaf, and more than one-third refused referral to a specialist. (These figures are comparable to those reported by Schlesinger, 1971.) Once a child reached an otologist (ear specialist) or special clinic with an audiologist, there were fewer diagnostic mistakes.

False hopes may be stimulated by the physician's refusal to accept a parent's suspicions, and some observations will probably support the hope of normality.

One of our resource people commented:

> Our experience has been that parents are generally reluctant, because of the social stigma attached or other reasons, to accept the possibility that their child may be deaf. Partly because a doctor may not be readily . . . available to them, and partly because confirmation of their own suspicions would be highly unpalatable, parents have a tendency to delay obtaining a firm diagnosis as long as there remain straws to be clutched at. Doubtless even in the most advanced countries there are many parents who fall into this category. [Tan Chin Guan, personal communication, 1980]

REACTIONS TO THE DIAGNOSIS

We have no entirely satisfactory studies of how parents are told that their child is deaf; reports are always filtered through parental memories and feelings about the experience. It is clear, however, that a significant proportion of parents are very dissatisfied with methods of informing (Schlesinger, 1971), and it seems unwise to assume that this is merely because the news is unwelcome. [Descriptions of parental reactions and what followed may be found in Pahz and Pahz (1977), Pfetzing (1971), and Spradley and Spradley (1978).]

Although a few parents deny the possibility of deafness in their child when they are given the diagnosis, almost all want to be told the truth as early as possible. We make this statement based not only upon our own experience, but upon many surveys of parents whose children have other kinds of disabilities.

Frustrations seem to fall into three major categories: 1) information was given with little compassion or support; 2) inadequate information was provided about what to do and where to go for help, or was not followed up and repeated as necessary; and 3) misleading information was given (such as advice to return when the child is older, or to have surgery that delays starting a necessary program).

One of our parent resource people wrote:

> I'm a mother who knew my child was deaf and was totally unsupported for 18 months. His first test was at 18 months of age; the hospital said nothing was wrong, yet at the test he didn't respond. The diagnosis was eventually changed to a central processing problem—also untrue. I am still angry at the professionals, particularly because, when confronted with evidence later, they refused to admit any error. . . . My major point is: believe the mother!

Few parents, it seems, obtain any sense of what life can be like for a deaf person from the early advice given— probably because the professional simply does not know.

Many writers have described fairly typical emotional reactions to the news that the child is handicapped: shock, denial, grief, anger, and guilt. Each parent is different, but some kind of strong reaction is common. One parent may blame the other. They may take their child to several professionals for re-testing, and may even perform repeated informal tests themselves, hoping that the diagnosis is wrong. A mixture of questions seems common: "Why has this happened to me? What did I do to cause it? How can I ever cope with it?" Many parents find it difficult to understand why it may be difficult or impossible to specify the cause. They may wonder whether it is possible for their deaf child to grow up to live a happy, fulfilling life without curing or bypassing the hearing loss. Hopes may be demolished without anything to replace them.

Other questions may return to plague parents: "How will he know that I love him? How will I discipline him? What will others think? How can I explain?" The months following diagnosis are a particularly vulnerable time for most hearing parents. They may feel isolated and alone. Much of the pain seems to arise because of a frustrating search for meaning, purpose, and communication. It is difficult to live with your deaf child day by day, knowing that something is wrong, but not knowing what the implications are or what to do about it. Fearing the worst, it is difficult at the same time to develop and nourish an emotional bond.

The diagnosis of a chronic disability always has unique individual significance for a parent, because its perception is partly influenced by past experiences that may include having a person with a disability in the family, being teased by other children because of some real or imagined peculiarity, or one's own successes or failures.

The adjustment to a major change in one's life typically results in disturbed and changeable emotions, the reawakening of unpleasant feelings from earlier times, and even physical changes in appetite, sleep patterns, and sexual behavior. What is worse, the reactions of mothers and fathers are often poorly matched to each other. They may then feel even more isolated, misunderstood, and deprived of joy. It is important to know that this painful process is normal, usually temporary, and not necessarily an indication of either mental illness or breakdown of the marriage.

It may surprise some workers in the field of deafness to learn that in the Vancouver study no significant increase in divorce or separation among the parents of deaf children was found (Freeman et al., 1975). Some parents with preexisting marital problems found that these were aggravated by the crisis of diagnosis; others reported that they were brought closer together. There is no single pattern; this is confirmed by studies of the families of children with other kinds of disabilities (Gath, 1978; Jan, Freeman, and Scott, 1977).

The preceding descriptions may seem to be very negative about professional shortcomings as seen by parents. Of course there are also parents who have received timely and compassionate help, and this should be acknowledged while efforts are made for improvements in professional training.

In addition, the statements made about parental emotional reactions are very general and need some balance. In the Vancouver study, parental guilt was much less prominent than we expected from reports in the literature. This was also reported by Schwirian (1976), although the fact that rubella was usually the identified cause in the latter study may have affected the findings. The point is that prolonged guilt need not be a consequence of having a deaf child.

IMPORTANCE OF GRANDPARENTS

For many children and parents, grandparents are an important resource. They should be aware of professionals' advice so that they can be supportive. Parents of a young deaf child often feel helpless at first, and may tend to fall back more on their own parents for comfort and assistance. Although there are situations in which grandparents find it very difficult to accept the deafness and continue to interfere in its management, it is likely that in most instances they have not been fully informed, nor have their own feelings and attitudes been considered. We strongly recommend that, if you are having difficulty with your own parents in relation to your child's deafness, you try to bring them into the picture with the assistance of those persons who are helping you.

HOW CAN THE IMPACT OF THE DIAGNOSIS BE REDUCED?

1. Parental concerns should be taken seriously. This requires better training of physicians and others involved in screening programs and in diagnosis—something parent groups can encourage.
2. Parents should have earlier counseling about deafness, including contact with other parents and with deaf people. (This will help to eliminate one basis for suffering: false stereotypes and false impressions of deaf people.)
3. Parents should have a supportive relationship with at least one non-judgmental professional who can help them sort out their questions and worries and restore communication within the family. Although this person should ideally be an

expert on deafness, he or she could also be one with limited knowledge in the field, as long as the person is not afraid to admit it, knows how to listen, and can help parents find answers elsewhere.

4. There should be an early program both for the deaf child and for the parents; failing this, there should be substitute activities (some of which are described in Chapter 15).

5. The parents' reactions to the diagnosis need to be monitored. How are they adjusting emotionally to their deaf child and to each other? Do they need special help? (This monitoring needs to be done by someone with experience in reactions to loss.)

6. Physicians and audiologists should be informed when they have failed to make a correct diagnosis.

In offering these suggestions, we recognize that saying something "should" happen is not enough to bring it about, and that what can be done will vary from place to place.

SUMMARY

1. Parental observations are important in identifying hearing loss in young children.
2. To avoid a prolonged delay in starting a necessary program, physicians need to take parental concerns seriously.
3. Bad feelings of parents toward themselves, toward each other, toward their deaf child, or toward professionals can have unfortunate effects.
4. Many parents report dissatisfaction with how the diagnosis is given or with the nature of the information provided about life as a deaf person.
5. Although parental emotional reactions to the diagnosis are common, and indeed a necessary part of adjustment, they need not be a permanent problem; they can be minimized by proper information and counseling. Family breakdown is not more common in families that include a deaf child.

Chapter 4

HOW CAN YOU BE SURE?

I want to have it explained a bit more. I mean I know all about the inner ear, and the outer ear, but I want to know why Karl's deaf, whether it's a nerve or what. . . . I don't think they know quite whether it can be put right. I'm building my hopes, that it can be put right. . . . I would like to know on the medical side, can she have adenoids and tonsils out, will it help her with her speech? Is there an operation? No one ever seemed to look deeper. They just said she was deaf. . . . [Quotes from three English mothers, taken from Gregory, 1976, pp. 163–164]

INTRODUCTION

Unless a deaf person is wearing a clearly visible hearing aid or is using signing or fingerspelling to communicate, the difference from others is *invisible*. Nothing is revealed by the appearance of the external ear. It is therefore difficult to be sure that something is indeed wrong with the mysterious inner workings of your child's hearing mechanism.

Many parents have continuous questions about the process of hearing and about audiometric or hearing testing, even years after the diagnosis of deafness has been established.

This chapter is a brief overview of how the physician or audiologist can tell that a child is deaf and how one can determine the type and severity of hearing loss. This is a complex subject and there is unfortunately no way to simplify it for parents as much as we would like while retaining enough accuracy for professionals. Some parents may wish to skim this chapter, or they may find it necessary to read it more than once. We make no claim to present here sufficient information to satisfy everyone. There is no substitute for an expert who can take the time to relate the

answers to your questions to the specific situation of
your own child. (The use of hearing aids is covered in
Chapter 10.)

STRUCTURE OF THE EAR

The ear is divided into three major parts (see Figure 1): the
external ear (including both the fleshy part we see and the
external canal), the middle ear, and the inner ear.

The *external canal* conveys sound to the inside of the
skull through an opening in the temporal bone to the *eardrum*
or tympanic membrane. The lining of the canal produces
wax that normally helps protect the eardrum by moving
dead skin, dirt, and germs toward the outside. If too much
wax is produced or if it is too hard, hearing may be reduced
by blockage of the canal.

The eardrum is fully developed at birth (as are all parts
of the ear except the external ear) and is attached on its far
side to the *hammer* (or, in Latin, the "malleus"), the first of
a chain of the three tiniest bones in the body, known as
ossicles. When sound waves set the eardrum into motion,
the ossicles move, passing the vibration pattern across the
middle ear from the hammer through the *anvil* ("incus")
and *stirrup* ("stapes") to the *oval window*.

In the inner ear, sound must pass from air into liquid,
losing much of its energy, but fortunately the eardrum and
ossicles are designed to compensate for this. The footplate
of the stirrup covers the oval window, acting as a piston and
lever to set up waves in the fluid-filled *cochlea* of the inner
ear. The *round window*, shown in the diagram, has a flexible
covering that allows pressure waves to move back and forth
through the cochlea. The snail-shaped cochlea has two and
one-half coils, the largest of which is closest to the oval
window and is responsible for perception of the higher
frequency sounds.

The fluid of the cochlea, set in motion by the stirrup,
bends the *hair cells* (of which there are about 17,000) in each

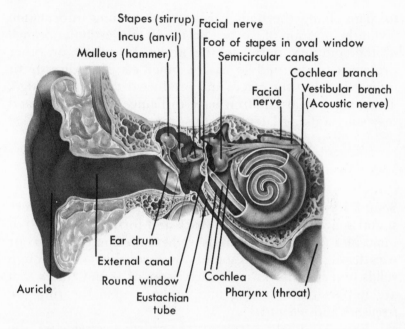

Figure 1. Structure of the ear. [Courtesy of Philips Electronics, Ltd., modified with permission.]

ear. When these are stimulated strongly enough, they generate an electrical impulse in the connecting nerve. These nerve impulses are then conveyed by the cochlear branch of the auditory nerve, via several complicated junctions, to the higher centers of the brain, where they are given meaning as perceived sound.

The middle ear is filled with air to keep the pressure equalized on both sides of the eardrum. This is accomplished by the *eustachian tube*, a ventilating canal connecting the middle ear to the throat. Air normally passes in and out by means of this tube when there are pressure changes; equalization is assisted by swallowing or yawning, and may be prevented by swelling (caused by infections, allergies, or enlarged adenoids).

The inner ear also contains the labyrinth, three fluid-filled *semi-circular canals* connected to the cochlea. They assist in maintaining the body's balance by sending information about the position of the head through the vestibular branch of the auditory nerve to the brain. Infections or other problems in the middle ear or inner ear may directly or indirectly affect the canals and produce dizziness or vertigo. Thus, some deaf children have difficulty with balance and may start walking later than the average child.

SOUND CONDUCTION

Sound waves move outward in all directions from every sound source by oscillations (back-and-forth movements) of molecules. Usually the sounds we hear are conducted to our ears through the air, but sound waves can also move through solids and liquids. Two characteristics of sound waves that are important in testing and understanding hearing are *frequency* and *intensity*.

Each complete oscillation is called a *cycle*, and the number of cycles generated by a sound source every second is known as its frequency. The abbreviation Hz is now used to represent cycles per second, in honor of Heinrich Hertz, one of the most famous scientists who studied sound. Thus, "50 Hz" means a frequency of 50 cycles per second. Human ears can normally detect sounds within a frequency range of 20 Hz to 20,000 Hz, and the speech range lies mostly between 100 Hz and 8,000 Hz. The higher the frequency, the higher the *pitch*, or tone, we hear. (For example, the lowest and highest "C" notes on a piano have frequencies of about 30 Hz and 2,050 Hz, respectively.) Almost all of the sounds that we hear are combinations of many frequencies, but some of the sounds used in hearing tests are of only a single frequency, and are known as *pure tones*.

Sound waves exert pressure on surfaces they contact; this can be used as a measure of a sound's *intensity* or power. The greater the intensity of the sound waves on our eardrums, the louder is the sound we hear. A sound that we are just able to hear is said to be at our *threshold* intensity.

(These definitions and explanations may seem very technical, but are important for understanding hearing tests.)

To compare the hearing of one person with another, it is essential to be able to measure the intensity of sounds that are heard. An arbitrary sound pressure level was agreed upon internationally as a reference point. This reference pressure corresponds approximately to that of our threshold intensity for a sound with a frequency of 1,000 Hz. Other sound pressures are compared to this reference pressure on a scale measured in *decibels* (abbreviated dB), a name derived from the inventor of the telephone, Alexander Graham Bell. (Contrary to what many people think, a loss measured in dB is *not* a percentage of hearing lost.) Sound intensities on this scale increase tenfold for every 20-dB difference in sound pressure. A sound pressure of 20 dB would roughly correspond to a whisper in loudness, and 140 dB would correspond to the loudness of a jet engine at take-off when you are about 100 feet (30 meters) from it.

Air conduction of sound (mentioned above) occurs via the external ear to the middle and inner ears. A blockage in the external or middle ears usually means an overall reduction in all sound intensities, but not a total hearing loss, because there is another route for sound—*bone conduction.* Sound vibrations are transmitted through the skull bones directly to the cochlea; this is partly how we hear our own voices. Hearing tests examine both routes: air conduction by earphones, and bone conduction by means of a vibrating device placed on the forehead or on the mastoid bone behind the ear. If a person can hear better by bone than by air conduction, there is probably a loss caused by some obstruction in the conductive pathway, such as that caused by middle ear disease.

TESTING OF HEARING

Who tests hearing? Although general practitioners or pediatricians may test it in the office, their tests can be expected to give only a very crude and unreliable result. Far better results are obtained from two kinds of experts on hearing who cooperate on diagnosis and treatment: the audiologist and the otologist.

The *audiologist* is a non-medical professional with a Master's or Doctorate degree who is trained to evaluate hearing and who should be knowledgeable about types of loss and their management.

The *otologist* (or otolaryngologist) is a surgeon specializing in the diagnosis and treatment of diseases of the ear and of related parts of the body. The otologist's field is sometimes referred to as "ENT," standing for "Ear, Nose, and Throat." Otologists may make their own audiograms or depend upon an audiologist's findings.

At present only a few audiologists and otologists are familiar with the social and communicative aspects of deafness. It is to be hoped that their training will include these vital topics in the future.

Although *speech pathologists* may also have qualifications in audiology and may be very helpful with deaf children's speech, it should not be expected that all of them will be experts on deafness.

As the child develops, different tests are appropriate. In the first year of life we do not expect cooperation, or a response to spoken words, because the baby cannot fully appreciate what response is expected. (There are recently developed screening tests, such as the Crib-o-Gram, which can be used in the hospital newborn or intensive care nurseries to identify babies who may have a hearing loss. These tests are still being evaluated and are not yet in general use.) Newborns do not respond to soft sounds, such as whispers, but after babies are a few weeks old, a noise, music, or speech may cause a change in behavior, such as a startle, a movement of the head, or a change in activity. Measuring this response is still not accurate and gives only a very gross picture of the baby's hearing. By 12 months we expect the child to localize interesting sounds of different pitch. If the child has enough hearing, speech-hearing levels can be obtained between 15 and 30 months for both air and bone conduction, and some *conditioning* procedures may be successful. In a conditioning test, a loud sound is paired with the presentation of something that is visually interesting to the baby; after a number of repetitions the baby will "condition" or respond to the sound alone. The sound can then be progressively reduced in intensity and used for testing. A series of practice sessions may be needed.

Earphones may not be accepted by the young child. It may be necessary to present sounds without them, to both ears at once, in what is called *soundfield testing*. By 30 months, conditioning to pure tones is often possible. When full cooperation can be obtained, earphones can be used and formal audiometry can be completed.

An *audiogram* is a chart of the examiner's findings under several conditions: pure tone responses at a level that can barely be heard (threshold); tests for both ears separately by air conduction and bone conduction at different frequencies; and *speech reception thresholds*, or SRT. A pure tone test checks the *awareness* of a sound, not whether the child attaches meaning to speech at that level. The SRT is an indication of meaning perception; it is a measure of the minimum hearing level necessary to correctly identify 50% of the recorded words presented (this is an oversimplified definition). For assistance in prescribing a hearing aid, other determinations are also made, such as the most comfortable level of amplification and the highest level of tolerance (when the sound becomes painful). Another important test is for *speech discrimination ability*, which assesses whether the child can distinguish among various vowel and consonant sounds. When there is a large difference between the hearing thresholds of the two ears, it is necessary to prevent the better ear from responding and giving a false reading while the poorer ear is tested; this is done by "masking" the better ear (through the earphone) with a band of noise at about the same frequency as that being tested.

There are limitations to the tests we have described. All must be done in a soundproof booth or room. Those involving speech may not be helpful for a deaf child who has never heard sufficient undistorted speech to attach meaning to it. The child with a behavior problem or with additional physical impairment may be very difficult or impossible to test reliably. Repeated attempts may be necessary. There are also some special tests that can be given, which are described later in this book.

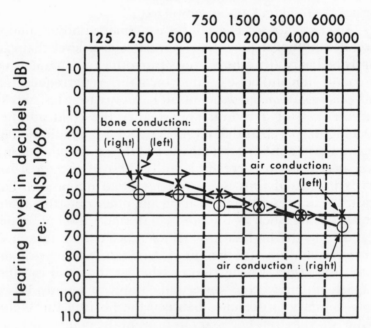

Figure 2. Sample audiogram (moderate sensorineural impairment). [Courtesy of George Muller.]

The audiogram (see Figure 2) is a graph with numbers representing frequencies (125 Hz to 8,000 Hz) listed horizontally and the hearing level in decibels (dB) listed vertically. As thresholds are determined for each frequency, a symbol is placed on the audiogram at a point where the frequency and hearing level intersect. (Red markings are used for the right ear, black or blue for the left ear; these colors are not shown on our figures.) Symbols used for air-conduction testing with earphones are "O" for the right ear and "X" for the left. Arrows open on the right ("<") represent bone conduction for the right ear; (">") represent conduction for the left. Symbols for air conduction are usually connected to make the hearing pattern readily visible. Special additional symbols are used when masking is employed. (See Lloyd and Kaplan, 1978, for a full guide to audiograms.)

Responses in the range of 0–25 dB are considered normal for children. Ordinary conversation takes place at about 40–50 dB, and those with normal hearing find levels of 125–140 dB painful.

There are many ways to refer to levels of severity of hearing loss. The one we have used, popular in North America, classes the children we are discussing as *profoundly deaf* if they have a loss of 91 dB or more, or *severely deaf* if their loss is between 71 dB and 90 dB. These figures are arrived at by taking the average of the most important speech frequencies for the better ear (usually 500, 1,000, and 2,000 Hz).

The tests previously described involve observations of the behavior of an alert and cooperative child. The relationship with the examiner is therefore very important. There are now other tests that require little or no cooperation and are especially useful for children who are difficult to test. These include the tests described below.

Impedance Audiometry

Impedance is a measure of the difficulty encountered in transferring sound energy from the external ear through the middle ear to the cochlea. Impedance audiometry procedures test the response of the eardrum, ossicles, and small muscles attached to the ossicles. Small, painless pressures are exerted in the external canal using a probe and an airtight seal, while different frequencies of sounds are reflected off the eardrum and the pattern is recorded. Eustachian tube function can also be evaluated by having the child swallow. A further part of the test is the use of a loud sound to produce a reflex contraction of a small muscle in the middle ear that stiffens the chain of ossicles to protect the inner ear (this is the *acoustic reflex*). Some information about sensorineural losses may be obtained from impedance testing if middle ear function is found to be normal after the age of about 5 months. These tests have several advantages: it is not usually necessary to sedate the child, a physician's presence is unnecessary, and a soundproof area is not required.

Auditory Brain Stem Response (ABR)

As the nerve impulses are passing through the lower levels of the brain from the auditory nerve on their way to the higher centers, they make connections in the brain stem, which is located near the base of the skull. Electrical activity (similar to the brain-wave test or EEG) can be recorded here by auditory brain stem response. The child is made sleepy or actually put to sleep with sedation so that cooperation and mental state do not affect the test results. Clicks or tone pips are fed into the child's ear, and a computer analyzes the results to tell whether the brain activity changes. This is not truly a test of the entire process of "hearing"—rather it helps to determine whether auditory signals are reaching the brain. The usefulness of this procedure with very young infants is not proven. It is not practical as a routine test because of the complex apparatus, the necessity of a physician's presence for sedation, and the cost. (This procedure is still not available everywhere.)

These "objective" tests (as well as others not described here, such as electrocochleography), may be especially useful for difficult-to-test or multiply-impaired children. For the professional interested in more details, the discussions of Martin (1978) and Northern and Downs (1978) are especially helpful. At present, it appears that impedance testing is the most widely applicable of these tests and that deaf children should be checked regularly by this technique.

Screening tests of hearing, useful for all children, or for children who are felt to be at higher risk for a hearing loss (such as those who are born prematurely), have been well discussed by Northern and Downs (1978).

All tests of hearing need to be combined with the child's history, with physical examination, and with other studies before a confident and comprehensive diagnosis can be achieved. Diagnostic tests should not be used in isolation, although after diagnosis some of them may be repeated without using the others.

TYPES OF HEARING LOSS

In *conductive* losses, sound is not well transmitted to the inner ear, but there is no distortion. Amplification and louder speech may help considerably. Surgical or medical treatment may also be very effective. The problem is only a mechanical one, because the delicate inner ear is normal. The intensities of all frequencies are reduced, but the loss is never much greater than 60 dB, because at that level the sounds bypass the middle ear by bone conduction. Causes of conductive losses include malformed ears (a congenital defect), infection, allergies, injuries, and wax plugs in the external ear.

Although none of the deaf children we are discussing have pure conductive losses, some attention to these problems is necessary because they occur so frequently in all children, and because they may reduce residual hearing in deaf children.

Earache is usually caused by acute otitis media, or a middle ear infection. The infection enters through the eustachian tube or through a perforated eardrum; fluid and pus build up, pressing against the drum and causing pain. If the infection is allowed to continue without treatment, the eardrum and ossicles may be damaged, or nearby mastoid bone may be invaded by the infection. When the otitis media becomes chronic, the ossicles may be destroyed.

A common childhood condition is popularly known as "glue ears," or, medically, as *serous otitis media*. There is no infection, but fluid ("serum") develops and thickens to the consistency of glue in the middle ear, making it difficult for the eardrum to move and thus reducing hearing. The cause may be a subsiding infection, or a reduction in ventilation of the middle ear because of blockage of the eustachian tube from swelling, caused by allergy or by enlarged adenoid tissue. If treatment to reduce the blockage of the eustachian tube is not successful, the eardrum must be lanced (*myringotomy*) and the fluid sucked out (*paracentesis*). Sometimes a plastic tube or grommet is inserted in the eardrum for several months to permit normal ventilation of the middle ear.

Sensory-neural Losses

Sensory-neural losses are what affect the children discussed in this book. They are caused by disorders of the cochlea or of the auditory nerve. Unlike conductive losses, sensory-neural losses affect not only loudness but also *fidelity*. This means that the sounds, when heard, are distorted. Voices may be heard but not understood, even with amplification. If the sensory-neural loss is present from early life, it is very difficult to use the distorted amplified sounds to learn to understand speech. Raising your voice to a person with a sensory-neural loss may not help. One of the most common patterns is loss of the high tones. (Recall that these sounds are perceived by the hair cells in the basal turn of the cochlea, the part nearest the middle ear, and therefore most likely to be damaged.)

Vowel sounds are low-pitched, and so they may be heard, but without the high-pitched consonants like "t," "k," and "p," words cannot be easily discriminated from each other.

Another feature of sensory-neural losses is that, as sounds build up in intensity, there may be a sudden increase in perceived loudness to the point at which it is painful. This is known as *recruitment*, and can make amplification and tolerance of noisy situations difficult. Ringing, buzzing, or roaring noises in the head, known as *tinnitus*, are common in adults, but seem less troublesome to deaf children. The cause is not well understood.

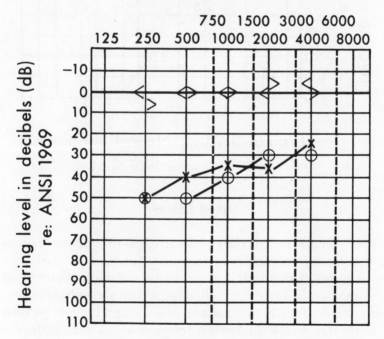

PURE TONE AUDIOGRAM
Frequency in Hertz (Hz)

Typical Conductive Impairment

Figure 3. Typical conductive impairment. [Courtesy of George Muller.]

PURE TONE AUDIOGRAM
Frequency in Hertz (Hz)

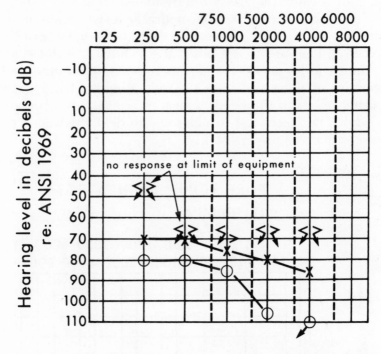

Typical Sensory-Neural Impairment

Figure 4. Typical sensory-neural impairment. [Courtesy of George Muller.]

Mixed Losses

Mixed losses also occur; the conductive loss may be permanent or temporary (as with recurrent infections).

Figures 3 through 5 show three common patterns of hearing loss. In Figure 3, indicating a typical conductive loss, bone conduction is normal and the air-conduction pattern is fairly flat across the speech frequencies. A very different pattern appears in Figure 4. In this sensory-neural loss, the bone conduction graph follows air conduction, indicating that both types of hearing are affected by cochlear or by

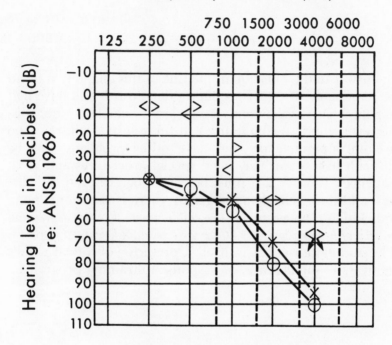

PURE TONE AUDIOGRAM
Frequency in Hertz (Hz)

Typical Mixed Impairment

Figure 5.   Typical mixed impairment. [Courtesy of George Muller.]

auditory nerve damage. Figure 5 shows a mixed pattern: bone conduction is better than air conduction, indicating a conductive problem, but the paralleling of the air-conduction line shows that both types of loss are present.

PROGRESSIVE HEARING LOSS

Progressive losses are those that continuously and significantly worsen over time; they are relatively rare. A treatment is very seldom available. Repeated testing is important in order to help the child and parents to understand what is happening, to plan for the future, and (in some instances) to seek genetic counseling.

CONCLUSIONS

In answer to the question in the title of this chapter, you can be reasonably sure of your child's diagnosis if you have had a competent assessment. Tests are available to do this; however, there are limitations to these tests. Children who are uncooperative or who have other problems may be difficult to test and may need special procedures and great patience. Another fact must be remembered: even with the best and most reliable audiograms, there is variation among individuals. *This means that two children with the same degree and pattern of hearing loss may utilize their residual hearing differently.* The audiogram is not in itself a predictor of a deaf child's motivation, intelligence, or response to training programs.

SUMMARY

1. The ear is an amazing mechanism for converting patterns of sound energy into electrical energy (nerve impulses) that can be given meaning when received by the brain.
2. Damage to the middle ear (conductive loss) reduces the message reaching the inner ear but does not eliminate it completely. Loud sounds can bypass the middle ear and go directly to the inner ear by bone conduction or can override the loss present.
3. Severe or profound deafness can occur only if there is damage to the cochlea or to the auditory nerve (i.e., sensory-neural deafness). Mixed impairments are not uncommon.
4. Conductive losses are often correctable; sensory-neural losses are rarely so.
5. Testing of hearing involves taking into account the child's developmental level, behavior, history, and physical examination, as well as other special tests. New tests have recently been developed for infant screening and for uncooperative, very young, and multiply impaired children.
6. Audiograms are detailed records of hearing tests. They include: pure tones, hearing for speech, speech discrimination, and others.
7. Other tests that are more objective and that require less cooperation include impedance testing of the middle ear and auditory brain stem responses.
8. The pattern of test results usually can give a very accurate report of the type of deafness and whether it can be treated. However, no test can predict how well the child will use residual hearing.
9. The interpretation of the tests and its translation into a program for the child is a much more complex and uncertain effort than merely reading an audiogram. Mature clinical judgment and input from several different disciplines are essential.

Chapter 5

WHY DID DEAFNESS HAPPEN?

WHY PARENTS WANT TO KNOW

Producing a normal child is an important parental need. The motives may include biological instinct (preservation of mankind), self-esteem, social pressures, a wish to care for and nurture someone younger and more helpless, a wish to continue the family line, a desire to prove that one is competent, a need to undo one's own bad experiences as a child, and many others. The effect of a child's deafness on the family needs to be understood in light of these emotionally loaded motives.

Aside from the obvious reason that knowing the cause of their child's deafness may influence how he or she is managed, parents (like all people) have a need to understand, and if possible to control, what happens to them. After the shock of diagnosis, parents often fear that in some way they have caused the deafness. These parental fears roughly fall into two categories: things they might have done wrong, and things they may have neglected to do. For example, those parents who emotionally rejected their child during the pregnancy (smoked too much, drank too much, engaged in sexual activity outside the times pronounced safe by their doctors, or tried to abort the unborn child), may feel guilty, although it is highly unlikely that any of these factors influenced the deafness.

Many parents blame themselves for circumstances over which they had no control. For instance:

> Our daughter was deafened by rubella—exposed during Louise's pregnancy while we were on a summer vacation. We blamed ourselves for taking that vacation, as though we should have somehow known that this was going to happen. Parents must be reassured that we have very little control over the circumstances that give rise to deafness in a child. [T. Spradley, personal communication, 1980]

Producing a child who is physically different often prompts feelings of inadequacy, especially if it is the first child. Knowing the cause of deafness is desirable and may help reduce doubts about the ability to cope with the loss.

Some families are very concerned with the question of genetics: which side of the family did it come from? Will the hereditary tendency affect others in the family who may not yet be born—the brothers and sisters of this deaf child? These are questions that should be answered for the family by their physician or, if the situation is complex, by referral to a genetic counseling clinic.

One mother whose child's deafness is thought to be genetic wrote to us:

> This was the most important and trying part of my personal encounter with deafness, and the time when I needed the most help. It is difficult to understand, unless you have been through it, just how important it suddenly becomes that you *must* know why, almost as if we all need to know that it was *not our fault*.

DOES KNOWING THE CAUSE MAKE ANY DIFFERENCE?

Beyond feelings of guilt, it may be important to identify a particular cause of deafness in order to provide more effective management. This may allow better planning for the child with a progressive hearing loss or with other physical defects associated with the deafness (Chapter 7), or for genetic counseling.

Knowing the cause may also be important psychologically, to help work out unrealistic feelings of guilt. Knowing the exact cause, and therefore knowing the magnitude of the risk of recurrence, make it easier to decide whether to take the risk of having another deaf child. The opportunity to discuss your ideas and doubts may be very helpful, whether or not a specific cause can be identified.

If distress about the cause of deafness continues, in spite of access to the best information available and sufficient opportunity for discussion, it is worth looking into the particular meaning that deafness may have for the family.

CAUSES OF SENSORY-NEURAL DEAFNESS

Introduction

If you still have questions about the causes of deafness, this discussion of sensory-neural deafness may be useful for you. If, on the other hand, the issue is well settled for you, you may wish to bypass this chapter.

We have tried to present sufficient information to satisfy most parents, but no brief description can do full justice to all kinds of situations. Further questions may be stimulated by the information given here. These questions should properly be taken up with the physician who best knows your child's situation. More space has been given to genetic causes of deafness than to other causes, simply because they are more difficult to understand and often arouse more family concern.

We have chosen just three broad categories by which to organize the complicated subject of deafness: 1) *acquired* or *environmental causes* that affected the baby *after* conception, 2) *hereditary* and *genetic causes* that took effect *at* conception, and 3) *unidentified causes*.

There are several sources of confusion: 1) deafness present at birth (congenital) can be acquired *or* genetic, 2) a genetic cause may result in deafness that has its onset after birth, 3) several causes may be operating together, and 4) environmental causes can sometimes mimic genetic causes.

There is no point in giving frequencies for each type of deafness, because they are often variable depending on when and where the study was done, on the severity of hearing impairment, and on the definitions used.

Knowledge of this field is developing rapidly, so this brief description should not be taken as conclusive.

Acquired or Environmental Causes

There are a few *ototoxic* (ear-damaging) drugs that can damage the baby's hearing either before or after birth; these include certain antibiotics for the treatment of infections, taken by injection or by mouth. (No complete list can be given here because knowledge is constantly changing.) In various countries different drugs are in use, with different warnings, and consumer protection may be very inadequate. Physicians are supposed to be aware of ototoxic effects, but sometimes either a woman's pregnancy is not known at the time she takes the drug, the drug is not yet known to cause damage, or it is necessary to take it (in spite of the risk) because no other drug will be life-saving. A few of the antibiotics known to have ototoxic potential are streptomycin, gentamicin, kanamycin, and neomycin. (Neomycin may be safely used in the external ear canal or in the eye, but entails an ototoxic risk when taken by mouth or by injection.)

Infections used to be a major cause of deafness. The best known examples are *rubella* (German measles) or *cytomegalovirus infection* (in the pregnant mother) and *meningitis* (in the child). In rubella deafness, the pregnant woman has a mild, sometimes unnoticed, rash and a fever. There is a risk of deafness in about one-third of these women's children, especially if their infection occurs in the first few months of pregnancy. The deafness is likely to be more marked in the higher frequencies. (In some instances the child's deafness may be progressive because of the continued presence of the virus after birth.)

Cytomegalovirus infections are fairly common in pregnant women. Hearing impairment of varying severity is said to occur in up to half of infected children (Catlin, 1978).

Meningitis involves an infection and inflammation of the coverings of the brain and of the nerves that lead into it. Most meningitis occurs in children under the age of five. According to a recent study (Keane et al., 1979), about 6% of children with bacterial meningitis are left with a sensory-neural hearing impairment, although other investigators report a higher frequency of occurrence.

Another type of infection is toxoplasmosis, a generalized protozoan infection of the mother that can cause hearing impairment in 17% of infected children (Abrams, 1977).

There are several types of injury that can damage hearing. The most obvious is a fracture through the temporal bone of the skull, but damage may also occur from severe lack of oxygen during labor or delivery (such as from a short umbilical cord tightly wound around the neck), from severe prematurity (being born much too early), and from other causes. Another form of injury, now largely preventable, is *kernicterus*, or the depositing of bile pigments in the brain. If present in sufficient quantity, bile pigments not only cause jaundice (yellowing of the skin), but also may damage the sensitive parts of the brain that control hearing and the coordination of movement. The usual cause of kernicterus is Rhesus, or Rh, incompatibility. In this condition, the mother and baby have different blood types: the mother is Rh negative and the baby is Rh positive. After the mother becomes sensitized to the baby's red blood cells (usually during the second or later pregnancies), her body reacts against the baby's blood factor, producing antibodies that pass through the placenta and destroy the baby's red blood cells. This releases the bile pigments mentioned above. Rh-negative mothers can now be easily identified, and treatment is available to prevent or to modify the damage. As a result, few children born in developed countries suffer this type of deafness.

Hereditary or Genetic Causes

Most cases of genetic deafness are congenital and unchanging in severity. A minority, however, have a postnatal (after birth) onset and a few cases become more severe as the child grows older. Cotton (1977) reports that only eight out of 4,000 children examined had progressive deafness, although the definition of what constitutes significant worsening presents serious problems in comparing one study with another.

It is thought that the deafness of about half of all deaf children has a hereditary cause (although sometimes this cannot be proven). Over 90 types of genetic deafness have been identified (Konigsmark and Gorlin, 1976).

There are special problems in understanding genetic deafness, especially for parents who may not be familiar with the concepts or terms used. These need to be outlined before specific genetic mechanisms are explained.

How can we conclude that a person has deafness of genetic origin? In order to determine a genetic origin of deafness, the history of the child's deafness and health is investigated, medical records are obtained, a physical examination is performed (including the examination of any other physical features associated with the hearing loss), and any necessary additional tests are administered. The family health history is taken, and records and tests of family members may also be obtained. A pattern of physical features known to be associated with a hereditary form of deafness (a syndrome) may become evident, or a particular family "pedigree" of transmission of the deafness may emerge, or both may occur.

The experienced physician or genetic counselor may then consult the ever-expanding literature on specific syndromes. Sometimes a first-time occurrence of a type of hereditary deafness cannot be identified with confidence because of the lack of a family history; only when another case occurs in the family will sufficient information be available to make diagnosis certain.

Probability and the concept of "risk figures." Whether you have one son or five sons, the probability of your next child also being male is still one in two, or 50%. Similarly, if you have one deaf child, and the probability of having another (*recurrence risk*) is given as one in four, or 25%, this does *not* mean that the next three children will be hearing: the risk is one in four for *each subsequent* pregnancy, no matter what has happened with previous pregnancies. The past record of pregnancies is not relevant in this type of inherited pattern.

Characteristics inherited from each parent. Each child receives half of his or her genetic material from each parent. (The halves differ each time; if not, each child would be identical.) With one exception, all cells in the human body have 23 pairs of *chromosomes* (or a total of 46). Because the chromosomes are paired, each segment in one chromosome has a corresponding segment in its partner. It follows that *genes,* the actual units of inheritance, are also paired, one on each chromosome. The genes are a chemical coding system, strung like beads on a chain, which provides information for the development and functioning of various organ systems. At each gene location, the gene may take several forms: an individual may have two of the same genes, or one or both may be abnormal.

When the egg or sperm cells are being produced, the 46 chromosomes are divided into two sets of 23. This means that the egg and sperm cells that join at conception each have only 23 *unpaired* chromosomes. When they form the beginnings of a new human being, they combine to make the usual number of 46 chromosomes—23 from the mother and 23 from the father (one of each pair). Thus, each egg or sperm cell has only *one* copy of a particular gene.

A man produces many sperm; approximately half of them carry the gene from one of the paired chromosomes, and half from the other. The same is true of a woman's egg cells.

There are many different gene locations that control the complicated process of hearing, and many different varieties of genes that can occur at these locations. In different forms of deafness, different gene locations may be involved.

Tests for "carriers" and prenatal diagnosis.   There are very few specific tests at present to prove that a parent or a child is a carrier of a genetic disorder. This will undoubtedly change in the future, but for now it means that we must depend upon indirect evidence.

Most people are now aware of *amniocentesis*, the method of removing a small amount of fluid from the area surrounding the unborn child. The cells floating in it may then be tested to determine the child's sex and the presence or absence of certain developmental disorders. These tests are not yet useful in the diagnosis of deafness before birth.

Is it really genetic?   The physical picture usually associated with a genetic disorder can sometimes be mimicked by the picture produced by environmental factors (such as drugs, injuries, or infections). The results of different genetic disorders may look the same, or the results of one genetic disorder may produce very different clinical features. This is why an experienced worker in the field of human genetics may be needed to complete an investigation and to determine whether the disorder is really genetic. (The details of genetic mechanisms are described later in this chapter.)

Unidentified Causes

Depending upon the study, different researchers report that they are unable to identify a cause in 12%–50% of the cases of deafness in children. The reasons for this inability are difficult for many parents to understand. Probably a large proportion of these unidentified causes is genetic, but this cannot be proven because there is no family pattern. In other cases there simply is insufficient evidence. Physical changes seen on audiograms or x-rays are often non-specific: they do not usually indicate the cause of deafness.

Another source of confusion is the attribution of deafness to a known *possible* cause (such as an ototoxic drug) when it is not the *real* cause.

Causation may be difficult to determine. If there is continuing concern or confusion, it should be discussed with the physician and/or audiologist to see whether any further clarification is possible.

We have now briefly described three major classes of causes. Because the ways in which genetic mechanisms work are difficult to understand, we now discuss this area in greater detail. (Further technical information is available in Catlin, 1978; Cotton, 1977; Fraser, 1976; Holmes, 1977; Konigsmark and Gorlin, 1976; Nance and Sweeney, 1975; and Pashayan and Feingold, 1979.) Parents may find Fraser's chapter (1979), Kelly's book (1977), the booklets from Gallaudet College (1975), and the material from the National Foundation/March of Dimes (1980) helpful.

GENETIC MECHANISMS

Single Gene Defects

Autosomal recessive inheritance. Autosomal recessive inheritance accounts for 75%–80% of hereditary deafness. (The autosomes are all of the chromosomes other than the two sex chromosomes.) A type of gene that must be present in a double dose before deafness will result (both members of the gene pair must be of the same type) is known as *recessive*. In an affected person, both members of the gene pair must be of the abnormal variety. Both parents are usually normal and are not themselves affected. They are each carrying a recessive gene for deafness, but because the gene is present in only a single dose, it has no effect on them. Typically there is no family history of deafness, so a hereditary cause may be difficult for the family to understand. The risk of having a child with this type of genetic deafness is one in four, or 25% for each pregnancy, regardless of sex. (Reason: one in two of each parent's egg or sperm cells carries the gene for deafness; therefore, the chance of these two cells combining to produce a child with both deafness genes is one in two times one in two, or one in four.) The odds of having a child who is *not* a carrier are also one in four. The remainder (one in two) will be carriers like their parents, and will hear normally (see Figure 6).

The word "abnormal" often carries an emotional charge, but it simply means that a gene differs from the usual form and may produce a defect. For most hearing people, to be told that you are the carrier of an abnormal gene for deafness is a surprise and a shock, especially when there is no family history. However, geneticists have learned that we are *all* carriers of two or three abnormal genes that, if combined with another abnormal gene of the same kind from our spouse, would lead to an abnormal body structure or function in the child. The likelihood of this combination is very small, so we usually do not find out about it, and

Autosomal Recessive Inheritance

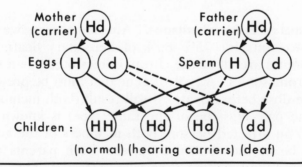

H = normal gene
d = faulty (recessive) gene for deafness

Figure 6. Autosomal recessive inheritance.

therefore wrongly assume that all our genes are normal. Relatives often have difficulty understanding the recessive mechanisms of inheritance and may need explanations from the professionals who are counseling the parents.

Sometimes two individuals whose deafness is of an autosomal recessive type marry and have children. If their deafness is caused by the same kind of abnormal genes, *all* their children will be deaf. If, however, deafness is caused by abnormal genes at different locations, all their children will be hearing; however, the children will all be carriers of two different deafness genes.

Autosomal dominant inheritance. The pattern of autosomal dominant inheritance accounts for about 20% of hereditary deafness. A variety of gene that is expressed if only *one* gene of the pair is present is said to be *dominant*. Typically the pattern is *generational*: at least one parent is deaf, and the deafness is seen in each generation, affecting approximately equal numbers of males and females. The risk of having another deaf child with this pattern is 50% if one parent has autosomal dominant deafness. (Reason: each child can get only a hearing gene from the hearing parent, and has a one in two, or 50%, chance of receiving the deafness gene from the deaf parent.) None of the hearing children will be carriers, because if they had the deafness gene, they would themselves be deaf. The children of these hearing children will have *no* increased risk of deafness (see Figure 7).

In the rare case in which both parents are deaf from the *same* autosomal dominant gene, there is a 75% chance of having a deaf child with each pregnancy, and a 25% chance of having a child who does not carry the gene. We can illustrate this by designating the dominant gene as "D" and the hearing gene as "h." The parents can each be shown as "Dh" and there will be four equally likely possibilities of combinations for their children to receive through the combination of Dh times Dh: DD, Dh, Dh, and hh. The first

Autosomal Dominant Inheritance

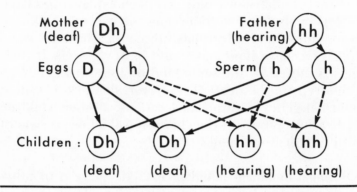

D = faulty (dominant) gene for deafness
h = normal gene

Figure 7. Autosomal dominant inheritance.

three patterns result in a deaf child, and the fourth in a hearing child, which gives an average of three in four deaf children.

There are a few additional factors that have to be taken into account in this type of inheritance. Sometimes the deafness gene arises anew as a change (*mutation*) in a sperm or egg cell, without any family history. (Once this has happened, it will have the same effects as if it had been passed down from previous generations.) In many dominant conditions, the expression of the deafness can be so variable that it is difficult to be sure of the pattern without careful study. (For example, one family member may be profoundly deaf, while another may have a mild hearing loss.)

X-linked inheritance. X-linked inheritance is an unusual cause of deafness. One of the pairs of chromosomes determines sex. A female has two X chromosomes in this pair, or an XX pattern. Males have one X and one Y chromosome, or an XY pattern. When the 46 chromosome pairs divide in making sperm, half of the resulting sperm cells will have an

X, half a Y. Males thus determine the sex of their children, because mothers can give their children only an X chromosome. In X-linked genetic disorders, the abnormal gene is located on the X chromosome. The females are ordinarily protected by having another normal gene on their other X chromosome. Their pattern could be written as X'X, with the X' indicating the chromosome with the gene for deafness on it. The male, having only one X, is not protected if he receives the abnormal gene: X'Y. Thus, females are carriers, and have a one in two chance of giving the X' to any one son (who will be deaf), and to any one daughter (who will be a carrier). Affected males cannot pass the deafness on to their sons, because they only give them the Y, but *all* their daughters will be carriers, because their daughters must receive their father's X' chromosome. The generational pattern is therefore a "skipped" one: normal (carrier) mothers may have deaf sons, but all the children of that deaf son will be apparently normal, and so on. (See Figure 8.)

X-Linked Inheritance

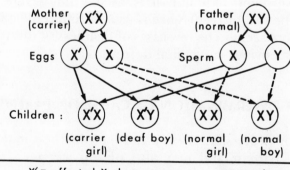

X' = affected X chromosome   XY = male
X = normal X chromosome   XX = female
X'Y = all his daughters will be carriers (they will get one
normal X from mother and must get the faulty X'
from their father); all his sons will be normal

Figure 8. X-linked inheritance.

Chromosomal Disorders

Sometimes, something goes wrong when the 46 chromosomes are being reduced to 23 in the formation of egg or
sperm cells. A chromosome may be broken, an extra one
may enter the cell, or one may be missing. Because many
genes are involved, a child born with this abnormality is
likely to have many serious defects. [This occurs about once
in 200 live births according to Holmes (1977).] The best
known example of a chromosomal disorder is Down Syndrome (commonly but wrongly known as "mongolism"), a
form of mental retardation associated with some degree of
hearing impairment in many children (Catlin, 1978). In rare
cases, these "genetic accidents" may be passed on to future
generations, but most are not. These special situations require individual genetic counseling.

Multifactorial Causes

More than one gene may be involved in causing hearing
impairment, with or without environmental influences. The
best example is cleft lip and/or palate, often associated with
hearing impairment, although it is usually not severe or
profound. The risk of recurrence is usually found to be less
than 5%. There seem to be few cases of deafness of this type
without other obvious congenital defects.

EFFECTS OF DETERMINATION OF CAUSE ON PARENTS

The search by professionals for a cause of deafness may be
confusing to parents and may also stir up worries about
additional defects not yet discovered.

There is no way to describe causes of deafness and
possible associated impairments without causing anxiety to
some parents. Only a competent physician with accsss to a
genetic counselor (when needed) can fully inform parents
regarding the causes of their own child's deafness.

Let us suppose that a hereditary cause has been ruled out or is unlikely. Does this mean that parents always stop worrying about the risk for future pregnancies? Not at all. Obviously you will be more anxious about future pregnancies if you already have a deaf child. Although there is about a 2% risk that *any* child will be born with a significant impairment of some sort, most parents simply do not worry much about it. When something *does* happen, the likelihood that there will be another problem looms much larger in their thinking. The worry spreads, but it is not necessarily in proportion to the actual risk. Such anxiety may even affect relatives or neighbors who are expecting babies.

One final point: sometimes a parent, anxious to know the cause of deafness, looks back on some event (such as an illness or injury) and believes that it really was the cause, in spite of advice from physicians that this belief is untrue. Parents may persist in this belief because of a need to reduce uncertainty and doubt, or because of feelings of guilt that cannot be reduced. In any case, such a belief is important only when it creates continuing problems.

OBTAINING GENETIC COUNSELING SERVICES

When a genetic cause is suspected, your physician and you may feel that a more complete and up-to-date investigation should be obtained from a qualified genetic counseling service. Genetic counseling is a communication process that deals with problems of the occurrence, or the risk of recurrence, of a genetic disorder in a family (Kelly, 1977). It can be helpful to parents who are trying to decide whether to have another child or who are concerned about the cause of the deafness, and to other family members who are worried about the risk for their future children. Genetic counseling can also help in identifying other associated health problems and in adding to research knowledge in order to benefit others.

In the past, such services were usually available only at university medical centers, but now they may be found at many non-university hospitals as well. Your physician or local agency for hearing-impaired children should know their locations.

If you are not completely clear about what you are told concerning your child's deafness, it may be a good idea to request that the information be summarized in writing, so that you can refer to it later or can show it to relatives or friends.

SUMMARY

1. There are many reasons why parents want to know (and should know) the cause of their child's deafness: *objective* reasons (hoping that it will help with management or will permit a wiser decision about having more children), and *subjective* reasons (needing to deal with guilt, self-doubt, a feeling of lack of control, or marital and family conflict).

2. About half the cases of deafness are thought to be "acquired" (caused by injury, infection, or drugs).

3. The remainder are probably of hereditary or genetic origin, but often cannot be proven to be so. These are briefly described as single-gene, chromosomal, or multifactorial in type. (Autosomal recessive inheritance is the most frequent genetic pattern.)

4. Genetic investigation and counseling are often helpful but must be highly individualized.

Chapter 6

CAN DEAFNESS BE CURED?

One of the well-known techniques for parental coping with the deaf child, once the deafness is discovered, is the hope for magical cures. Parents hope for operations, for new electronic gadgets, and for radical new teaching techniques. . . . All of these hopes have been exploited by various commercial and professional interests. [Mindel, 1971, p. 74]

Once a mother has come to terms with the fact that her child is deaf, very often she feels a very strong need for more explanation. What caused it? Is it curable? What about an operation? Many parents had always at the back of their minds the hope of a cure. [Gregory, 1976, p. 163]

INTRODUCTION

There is no cure for sensory-neural deafness; perhaps there will be some day. Why is it so difficult to accomplish? At least one reason is that the nerve connections within the inner ear (*cochlea*) and the auditory nerve are so complex that any surgical technique would have to make thousands of re-arrangements.

Why do many hearing parents continue to be interested in cures, even though they may know that none is possible? There are several reasons, perhaps different ones for each parent: 1) adjusting to a major change in expectations for the child is difficult and painful; 2) some professionals may encourage false hope; 3) relatives and friends are frequently on the lookout for reported cures, and have had even less opportunity than parents to deal with their own doubts and confusion; and 4) as hearing persons, parents cannot really imagine a successful and happy life without the ability to hear.

In this chapter, we briefly examine some of the recently reported methods of treatment or cure, sources of confusion about cure, reasons why overdependence on cure can be dangerous, and what can be done about the problems involved.

MIXED FORMS OF HEARING IMPAIRMENT

Middle ear disease (often causing a treatable conductive loss) tends to be common in young deaf children. Many deaf children, at one time or another, have middle ear infections, inflammation, or fluid behind the eardrum. The audiogram may then show a mixed type of hearing loss (conductive and sensory-neural). There are also special tests, such as the tympanogram, that the audiologist or otologist can administer to determine whether the eardrum is working normally (part of impedance audiometry—see Chapter 4). Without correcting middle ear disease, it may be hard to tell how severe the sensory-neural part of the hearing loss is. Because middle ear disease is often curable (but sensory-neural deafness is not), doctors and parents may hope that successful treatment of middle ear disease will cure or will substantially improve the total ability to hear.

There is no doubt that middle ear disease *should* be vigorously treated whenever it occurs; it can be dangerous to both general health and residual hearing. Sometimes this treatment delays the start of a much-needed educational program, although it should not.

NEW "CURES"

Research techniques are being tried that have been given much publicity, especially cochlear implants and acupuncture. All these methods have been (or are being) subjected to scientific evaluation and research (Linthicum, 1979). Undoubtedly more methods will be publicized from time to time. However, you should realize: 1) the unusual difficulties involved in "solving" this type of problem, 2) the temptation to be overly hopeful about any publicized "cures," and 3) the fact that preliminary research results are typically exaggerated by the media long before they have been thoroughly proven.

Acupuncture

Acupuncture has been used to treat deafness in the People's Republic of China and recently was tried in North America after political relations were re-established with that country. After initial enthusiasm, its popularity seems to have declined. There is no scientific evidence of its usefulness for sensory-neural deafness (Chasin, 1979).

Cochlear Implants

Cochlear implants are still being investigated. In this technique, developed in Australia, France, and the United States, very fine wires are placed in the cochlea and attached to an induction coil beneath the skin. Another coil outside the skin is attached to a stimulator activated by sound. Unfortunately, the cochlear implant, at its present state of development, does not enable prelingually deaf persons to understand connected speech or to attach meaning to speech sounds, although it does provide greater awareness of sounds. There are still many technical obstacles to overcome before implants will have any practical value; even then, many experts think that only postlingually deafened people may be helped.

Miracle Cures and Quackery

Many parents continue to search for, or be distracted by, "miracle cures" of a different type: either true religious miracles or forms of pseudo-scientific quackery not tested scientifically. Here is a description of the experience from one of our parent resource people:

> Relatives have a lot to do with the miracle cure stuff. It is a terrible burden. My sophisticated mother-in-law literally came sneaking into the house one day with a faith healer! This not only upset me badly (I was looked upon as cruel and insensitive when I refused him access), but was devastating in its implications. Clearly my mother-in-law thought of his deafness as an insurmountable tragedy— no help for a parent trying to cope! Relatives and friends come in the name of love, and their techniques often unconsciously involve emotional blackmail: reject my view, reject me.

DANGERS IN DEPENDING UPON CURES

There are real dangers when parents actively seek one miracle or medical cure after another: 1) normal and necessary grieving may be avoided, 2) false hope is reinforced, 3) there may be repeated disappointment and depression, and 4) the emotional attitude that deafness is a tragedy requiring a miracle (as illustrated above) is perpetuated. As a result of these excessive reactions, some parents fail to get on with the essential task of accepting their deaf child as a full member of the family. Perhaps an example from another field—blindness—can illustrate the point. For an older individual who becomes blind, or for parents of a blind child, the false hope of cure can be a disaster if it prevents (as it all too often does) working toward a normal and happy life as a *blind* person. Acceptance of blindness requires a commitment to learning new techniques of reading, of moving about, and of eating. Unfortunately, studies have shown that it is not unusual for eye doctors to avoid "hurting" patients or their families with the bad news that there is no hope for a cure of the blindness.

REDUCING DEPENDENCE UPON CURE

Many deaf children's parents find it impossible to stop hoping for a cure or to refrain from reacting with a surge of excitement to each newspaper article about deafness. Even if they try, this false hope is often encouraged by well-meaning friends, relatives, and new acquaintances when they learn about the child's deafness. There are some effective ways to help to reduce this tendency, although for most hearing people it may never be completely eliminated. We will explore one of them in this book: developing a new and realistic picture of deafness *as it is lived.* A second way is for you as a parent to maintain contact with a respected expert, or with a parent organization with professional advisers. Any significant discovery or method will then come to your attention without your having to sort everything out for yourself.

Perhaps the greatest forces that help to restore balance to a deaf child's family are learning to communicate and realizing that deaf children can develop normally.

CONCLUSION

Even though sensory-neural deafness cannot be cured, the hope of cure is a natural reaction of hearing parents (and their family and friends). This hope becomes an obstacle only when it is so powerful that it prevents the acceptance of the deaf child and the pursuit of a needed program. Miracles cannot be depended upon. There is no way to give up the excessive hope of cure without some pain and without restoring your pride in your deaf child. Taking positive steps to develop and improve communication and to share experiences and feelings with other hearing and deaf parents will usually help.

SUMMARY

1. The hope of cure is natural for hearing parents.
2. The dangers of excessive dependency upon the
   hope of cure are that it may waste time and
   money and may also prevent effective action that
   is necessary for the deaf child.
3. Middle ear disease may be mixed with sensory-
   neural deafness; sometimes parents or
   professionals hope that treating the middle ear
   will totally eliminate the problem. Deaf children
   seem to have more middle ear problems than
   children with normal hearing. These should
   always be treated, whether or not a "cure"
   results.
4. Publicity is frequently given to "miracle" cures,
   raising false hopes. Sometimes these cures are
   outright quackery; at other times legitimate
   scientific work is prematurely reported or the
   benefits are exaggerated.
5. Acupuncture has not been found to have any
   value in sensory-neural deafness.
6. Cochlear implants are still in an early research
   stage; they may eventually have real value for
   postlingually deafened individuals, but it is
   doubtful whether they will ever benefit children
   with sensory-neural deafness.

Chapter 7

ASSOCIATED PROBLEMS
What They Are and
What They're Not

Parents who are having difficulty accepting their child's deafness are sometimes shocked to learn that something else is also wrong including some form of brain damage (such as cerebral palsy), a heart defect, an eye problem, or suspected mental retardation. The combined impact can be overwhelming. Before overreacting, however, caution and a sense of perspective are advisable. The essential point to keep in mind is that a medical label need not always have practical significance, and even if it does, what is a problem to one person may not be a problem to another, or the importance of the problem may change over time.

The specific aspects of understanding and working with a multiply handicapped deaf child will be discussed in more detail in Chapter 22. At this point, we wish to introduce the general subject, and to show that additional impairments may not be as significant to a child's life as some parents fear.

The terms "impairment," "disability," and "handicap" are often used interchangeably, but there are useful distinctions to be made among them that we will try to maintain. *Impairment* refers to the actual physical or structural deviation from normal. It may have little or no practical consequence. All people who wear prescription eyeglasses have some visual impairment. Similarly, a mild hearing loss that is correctable by means of a hearing aid may result in few limitations. A *disability* refers to the loss of an important function in spite of any aids or treatment. Everyone who is disabled has an impairment, but not everyone with an impairment is disabled. If a hearing aid cannot correct for an impairment, and the person cannot perform an important function, this may be considered a disability. A *handicap* refers to attitudes, feelings, and barriers that increase the effects of a disability, turn it into a problem of living, and put a person at a disadvantage. A qualified deaf person who cannot obtain a job because of employer attitudes or because of the lack of a communication device on the telephone is handicapped. Another example of handicap is a person with epilepsy who is subject to repeated spells or seizures when he is off medication. When the condition is fully controlled by drugs, there is no disability. On the other hand, if the epileptic person desired to get married and was prevented by law (as was the case in certain areas until recently), then epilepsy would constitute a handicap.

These examples illustrate that the dividing line between these terms is not absolute. For a deaf person who signs, there is ordinarily no disability or handicap when he or she is with other deaf signers who use the same communication system (in spite of a hearing impairment). On the contrary, a hearing non signer is *disabled* when among deaf persons, and could be discriminated against (in which case non-signing would be a handicap).

The additional medical labels applied to some deaf children may represent impairments, not disabilities or handicaps. If a parent or teacher treats a deaf child as if there were an additional disability (such as mental retardation) when there is none, that child may be handicapped. A very good example of this was reported by Bergman and Stamm in 1967. They were interested in what happened to children in the Boston area who were said to have a heart defect or heart murmur. They discovered that many of the children with murmurs (which had no actual significance) had had their physical exercise restricted by parents or teachers. Their conclusion was that the unfounded fear of a heart attack caused more handicap than all the truly major heart conditions in children.

In fact, deaf children are more likely to have additional medical labels applied to them. Depending upon the survey, the type of deafness, and the severity of the additional impairment, the reported figures range from 11% to over 40%. (See Budden et al., 1974; Rawlings and Gentile, 1970; and Schein, 1974, for further details.)

The type of additional impairment depends partly upon the cause of the deafness. Rubella deaf children, of whom some 13%–60% are said to have additional impairments (Chess, Korn, and Fernandez, 1971; Peckham et al., 1979), are most likely to have cardiac defects, eye defects, or mental retardation. It is now known that many rubella deaf children have no additional defects, and that a history of infection with skin rash in the mother is often not obtained (Peckham et al., 1979). Mental retardation occurs in about 15% of children whose deafness is associated with meningitis. Rh blood incompatibility, producing severe jaundice and deafness, is associated with other physical impairments in about 75% of the children. Cerebral palsy is the most common additional diagnosis.

For each impairment in addition to deafness, there is a wide range of severity. For example, mild cerebral palsy may be of no consequence, except that a child may never become a well-coordinated athlete. Cardiac problems are often less important than parents imagine from their knowledge of adult cardiac disease. Visual impairment of some degree is considerably more common among deaf than among hearing children, and should be detected and corrected if at all possible because of the deaf child's dependence upon vision for communication.

Mental retardation is often hard to identify with confidence in a very young deaf child; if it is present, it may make it more difficult to specify the severity of hearing loss. Retardation may be suspected when progress in motor development or communication is slower than expected.

CONCLUSIONS

Deaf people with good ability have been misdiagnosed as mentally retarded; some with poor balance in childhood have been labeled as having cerebral palsy. Many of those with additional medical labels function very well. The challenge is not to reject a label, but to understand what the child can and cannot do, and then to see what can be achieved under the best possible circumstances.

SUMMARY

1. Medical labels other than deafness are more likely to be applied to deaf than to hearing children; these may not always have practical significance in everyday life or in school.
2. The terms "impairment," "disability," and "handicap" are sometimes used interchangeably, but it may be advantageous to distinguish among them, especially because these terms include a large social component that may be modifiable.
3. The frequency of additional impairments in deaf children is reported in different studies to range from 11% to more than 40%.
4. A very brief mention is made of the most frequent or important types of additional impairments; detailed discussion can be found in Chapter 22. Of particular significance is the frequency of visual impairment, often unrecognized, that may limit a deaf child's learning and attention.

Chapter 8
THE PARENTS' DILEMMA
What To Do

THE DILEMMA

When you have realized that your child is deaf and that he or she will continue to be deaf, you must make a decision about what to do concerning the child's development. Strong differences in professional opinion about various programs make this decision more difficult. Sometimes unrealistic publicity about the "success" of deaf children may lull parents into complacency:

> Parents, in fact, had little idea what they could hope for for their child in the future, and were unsure of the place their child might take in society. Most of them assumed that integration was the ideal, and a real possibility. [Gregory, 1976, p. 209]

This chapter examines the very different goals and the penalties involved in the basic decision that parents of deaf children must make in choosing between an oral-only and a Total Communication philosophy for their child's development.

THE ORAL-ONLY APPROACH

The goals of the oral-only approach are to enable the child to have the spoken language of the majority of people as a native language, to use it within the family and in school, and to eventually function normally in the "hearing world," with total integration being the ideal result. Intelligible speech is all-important, and is to be achieved by early amplification, by auditory training, and by speechreading. Signs and fingerspelling are forbidden, because they are considered dangerous for speech development.

The quotes that follow are from two brochures of the Alexander Graham Bell Association for the Deaf. The older one (undated, a) states that deaf people sign because "it is an easy way to communicate ideas" (p. 8). The child who is allowed to use all forms of communication "tend[s] to use only the manual forms; consequently his listening and speech suffer" (p. 9). The current undated brochure (undated, b) makes no mention of sign language, but declares without any restrictions: "He [the deaf child] will learn to communicate successfully with others through speech and hearing" (p. 1). In addition, the brochure makes the following suggestion:

> . . . talk to your child, knowing that by using his hearing aids he can hear you, and that through listening he will learn to develop speech through the same process as other children do. The normal learning process will take place with your child, but it is your responsibility to set the scene just right in order to compensate for the reduction in hearing ability. [pp. 7–8, emphasis from the original]

What happens to the majority of parents, for whom the promise of success for their child is not kept? The meaning seems clear to them: they have not done everything "just right"; but they should also ask themselves whether anyone could.

How is failure perceived by parents under the oral-only system? One reaction follows:

> For the first time I realized that we had worked so hard on speech and lip reading that we had never fully entertained the possibility of failure. In a few months Lynn would celebrate her fifth birthday. She could not talk; the few words she spoke were intelligible only to us and a few close friends. . . . What if all our efforts, what if all Lynn's valiant attempts actually did fail? What then? . . . the alternatives conjured up animalistic, nonhuman images in my mind. I feared to think of them. [Spradley and Spradley, 1978, p. 203]

The persisting hope for progress in speech, even after their child has failed, and the belief that sign language prevents progress can confuse and paralyze parents: "Several roads fanned out in front of us. All seemed to hold great risks for Lynn" (Spradley and Spradley, 1978, p. 221).

The strict oral-only approach makes several assumptions: 1) that life as a deaf person without intelligible speech and good speechreading skills is limited and failure-ridden; 2) that early and intensive auditory/oral training can lead to successful speech and speechreading development and absorption into "the hearing world" for most deaf children; and 3) that the additional use of sign language and fingerspelling will impair speech development. Additional but less fundamental assumptions are that spoken language is the "natural" language of deaf children and that it can be the "internal" language of thinking, that sign languages are not true languages, and that the early loss of easy two-way communication between parent and deaf child is not permanently damaging or very important. The actual problems of present-day deaf adults and teen-agers are discounted because it is argued that they did not have the benefits of modern techniques and equipment.

The oralists believe that, for deaf people, becoming like hearing people *can* be done and *must* be done, and that any other goal represents failure (Mindel and Vernon, 1971).

THE TOTAL COMMUNICATION APPROACH

The goal of the Total Communication approach is to use whatever means are available and suitable for an individual deaf child to develop (and to maintain) early communication both internally (thinking) and externally (with others). The means by which this is done are less important than the goal itself. Manual methods (sign language and fingerspelling) are added to auditory/oral methods from the earliest age possible. It is believed that whatever oral abilities the child has will become obvious at a later age and that these abilities are not hindered by signing. *Total Communication does not define success by speech intelligibility and speechreading alone; oral skills are considered valuable, but not all-important.* In addition, a comfortable social life should ordinarily involve the deaf person in the deaf community, and in whatever other circles he or she may choose.

The assumptions of Total Communication are: 1) that even with early auditory training, most deaf children, because of their hearing losses, will not be likely to develop intelligible speech that they can use as their primary means of communication; 2) that the inability to develop intelligible speech creates a situation that is dangerous because of the recognized need for some type of communication system in the earliest years; 3) that sign languages are perfectly good languages that can be acquired at the same rate as spoken languages; 4) that the use of a sign language or a signing system will not harm speech development if a quality Total Communication program is utilized; 5) that the experiences and views of deaf people are relevant—in fact, that deaf people need to be available as models for deaf children; and 6) that if families learn to sign, it will provide a natural and clear means of communication.

Total Communication advocates tend to operate according to a different value system than that of the oralists and to believe that trying to make the deaf child into a hearing child *cannot* be done and *need not* be done. The alternative situation—being a person who is different in some ways—is seen as an acceptable one.

[A recent, particularly good and readable account of the differing values and interpretations of the evidence involved in the controversy over methods of communication can be found in Benderly (*Psychology Today*, October, 1980).]

THE EVIDENCE

The following statements present evidence related to the oral-only and the Total Communication programs for deaf children:

1. Studies in Britain (Conrad, 1979) and in the U.S.A.
    (Jensema, Karchmer, and Trybus, 1978) show that by the

time most deaf children leave school (even in the *best* oral programs in Britain) they have not developed intelligible speech and are poor speechreaders.

2. Some of the few deaf children who *do* develop good speech have deaf parents and have signed as their first language. (This does not mean that early signing necessarily makes them better speakers, but it should demonstrate that signing does not have an automatically negative effect on speech development.) The language development of deaf children with hearing parents has also been followed carefully, and speech has improved while signing was used (Nordén, 1980; Schlesinger, 1978a; Schlesinger and Meadow, 1972).

3. Sign languages are full, satisfactory languages with a grammar of their own (Klima and Bellugi, 1979). Signs may also be used in the word order of a spoken language. Study of sign languages is still relatively new, but has been increasing at such a rapid rate in the last few years that many professionals and non-professionals in the field of deafness are not yet familiar with many of the advances that have been made (see Chapter 11).

4. Without an internal language (which may have neither audible sounds nor visible signs as its symbols), most deaf children are deprived of a means to develop their thinking, curiosity, socialization, and creativity at a time when their brains are most receptive (Conrad, 1979).

CONCLUSIONS

We strongly favor the Total Communication position as a result of our interpretation of recent evidence. It is our opinion that the oral-only approach involves unnecessary and dangerous risks, because of its concentration on what the child cannot do (and is not likely to do). A solid educational approach requires, instead, an emphasis upon what the deaf child *can* do, recognizing his or her strengths as well as weaknesses.

There is no way at present to predict which deaf children can be successful with an oral-only approach. Because sign languages have not been shown to affect negatively a child's

chances of developing good speech, it seems vitally important
to use signing as early as possible.

There are still many aspects of the use of non-speech
communication that need further study. The use of sign
language by deaf parents may have results different from its
use by hearing parents. We do not wish to suggest that sign
language is the answer to *all* the problems deaf children and
their families may have.

As a parent, making the "right" decision about your
child's future is an important step, but it is only a beginning.
Your responsibilities are not over when you pick the "right"
school or program. No matter what orientation you finally
believe is better for your child's communication, a considerable amount of continuing effort by you and your child
will still be necessary.

Even though a clear choice of different programs is not
available everywhere, it is still important to develop a positive
attitude toward non-speech communication and toward contact with deaf people. You may wish to make use of whatever
program is available (regardless of orientation) and to add
other components that you feel are necessary (described in
later chapters).

RECOMMENDATIONS

The following recommendations may help you in your choice
of a program:

1. Visit different programs and listen to different points of
    view, even if they are confusing at first. Be suspicious of any
    program that makes enormous promises; that minimizes the
    importance of your child's deafness, suggesting that it can be
    overcome; that advocates one perfect method of
    communication for all children; that exaggerates (or ignores)
    the usefulness of hearing aids for profoundly deaf children;
    or that suggests that deaf children can, in general, be fully
    integrated with hearing children.

2. Meet with deaf adults and children to modify any prejudices you may have. They have an essential contribution to make to your understanding of your deaf child. (Some ideas about how to meet with deaf persons are presented in Chapter 14. This is not a simple recommendation, because deaf persons may have their own prejudices and negative attitudes; therefore, a guided experience is advisable.)
3. Meet with other parents, especially those who have older deaf children. Include deaf parents of deaf children in these contacts.
4. Consider whether embarrassment for yourself or for your child when you are seen using hands in communication is influencing you. (Unintelligible vocalizations may draw even more attention.)
5. Consider whether any unpleasant childhood experiences you yourself may have had (being teased or being seen as "different") are influencing your decision.

SUMMARY

1. Opposing professional opinions about
    communication programs make parental decisions
    more difficult.
2. In an oral-only program, it is assumed that deaf
    children can, and indeed must acquire a spoken
    language as their native language, and that this
    necessary process is retarded or prevented by the
    use of signing or sign language. The deaf child's
    lack of early communication within the family is
    not believed to be significant enough to alter the
    emphasis on spoken language acquisition. It is
    viewed as unfortunate for a deaf child to grow up
    associating, by preference, mostly with other deaf
    people. Sweeping claims of success achieved by
    oralist methods are still being made without any
    statement of the proportion of failures.
3. Evidence does not support the claims for oral-only
    success (quite the reverse), nor has the use of
    signing or sign language been shown to prevent
    the development or use of speech.
4. Those advocating a Total Communication
    approach do not define success by looking at
    speech and speechreading alone—greater value is
    put on the early development of language and
    thinking (in any form) through two-way
    communication. All means of communication are
    encouraged so that the deaf child can participate
    as fully as possible in family life. It is the child's
    abilities that eventually decide what different
    means of communication are most suitable.
5. All issues are not yet settled, but there is evidence
    that best supports a flexible Total Communication
    approach. Parents should be exposed to different
    points of view and should understand the value of
    various programs and the evidence involved,
    because ultimately the responsibility for the deaf
    child is theirs.

Chapter 9
EARLY TWO-WAY COMMUNICATION

INTRODUCTION

When 108 English mothers of deaf children were interviewed for Gregory's (1976) study, they were asked what they felt their greatest problem was:

> . . . Seventy-six per cent of them gave answers indicating problems that arose from difficulties in communicating. When asked what they felt was the greatest problem from the child's point of view, 89 per cent replied that it was communication. [p. 20]

Gregory also gives a good description of what communication problems can be like in everyday life:

> What has emerged in our picture of the deaf child is that to some extent he lives in a segmented world. Continuity is lacking . . . because he has not the language to communicate and this has deep implications, not only for his present behaviour but also for his understanding of events and his ability to anticipate the future. One mother described how she watched her three children preparing for Christmas—making cards, hanging up decorations, and so forth. All of them were happy and excited, but whereas her two hearing daughters experienced it all as leading up to a climax on Christmas day, her deaf daughter could not properly appreciate what was going on or anticipate how it would come to a natural end. After Christmas she was unhappy, wanted to re-wrap the presents, to continue to make cards; the structure of the whole situation had been missing for her. [p. 205]

Aside from great difficulties in daily family life and limitations in understanding the social world, there are other reasons for concern about the development of early communication between deaf children and their families. Parents are often frustrated, and the desire for the child to speak and to understand speech may be so intense that it obscures the real risk of failing to develop any communication.

91

The very fact that deaf children seem to "get by" for several years under less than adequate circumstances can be deceptive.

In spite of considerable progress in the past 15 to 20 years, there is still much about language development that is mysterious. This chapter outlines a few of the facts and theories about language that relate to deaf children. We hope that this will help parents to appreciate later discussions on the different forms and functions of language.

WHAT IS COMMUNICATION?

"Communication" is a broader term than "language," and might be defined as any behavior that involves the sending and receiving of information between two organisms. For instance, insects and plants communicate with each other, and human beings communicate with other animals. Language is one vehicle for communication.

WHAT IS LANGUAGE?

What do we mean by a *language*? There is no completely satisfactory definition that everyone agrees upon, but there are certain characteristics of language as a communication system that we can outline:

1. *Language is systematic*. Elements recur in regular and meaningful patterns. Most sentences used are not memorized. They are created according to rules that the users share.
2. *Language is symbolic*. In many ways, language is an arbitrary code. Changing our experiences into words (spoken and written) or signs is called *encoding*. Signing, talking, and writing are different ways of *transmitting* these encoded messages. The recipient of these messages must then *decode* them back into the experiences that we are trying to share. This process implies abstraction: one or more words (or symbols, such as signs) stand for an event, a thing, a feeling,

or a concept that does not directly resemble what is referred to, including those things that are not present, or bound to the here and now. For example:

Mary watched silently as her husband John flopped into his easy chair and dis-appeared behind the newspaper. Anger was building up inside her and it suddenly exploded into words: "Don't you *care* at all about what *I've* been doing all day?" John looked up in surprise: "What are you mad about now?"

Mary transmitted her message in several ways; she expressed her feelings with words, with facial expression, and with tone of voice, all examples of the encoding of experience. John has obviously decoded all or most of these messages; at least he knows she is mad!

3. *Language is social, learned, and modified by experience.* Therefore, it reflects the requirements of the society using it.
4. *Language has a grammar.* The rules of grammar represent the formal features or structures that express relationships among words (or signs) and sentences. Each language has a grammar that is unique. When comparing various languages, both similarities and differences can be found.
5. *Language has meaning.* Connotations of words often go beyond dictionary listings. Different ways of thinking and being are reflected in the language of the culture using it. Gestures, intonation, and facial expressions accompany language (non-verbal communication), help in the understanding and enriching of communication, and differ from one language community to another.
6. *Language is variable.* Each individual uses language in a unique way, but those who share many similar experiences from early life on will have very similar usages. Systematic differences in pronunciation and vocabulary are referred to as dialect. All languages have dialects that are equally systematic and equally capable of further development. Dialects are not imperfect attempts at imitating a "real" or "ideal" standard form of the language, no matter what their social status. As a term used by linguists, "dialect" has no negative overtones. Everyone is a dialect user.
7. *Language evolves and changes.* The development process is slow and inevitable (unless all native users of the language are dead, as with Latin). Trying to preserve the form of language is futile, although complaints that English is

deteriorating have been expressed for centuries. Daily communication requires that language change as the people who use it develop new ideas and technology.

8. *Language can be communicated in a number of forms or modalities.* The most common vehicles are speech and hearing. Reading and writing are other modalities through which a spoken language can be adequately, though not always exactly, transmitted. Language can also be communicated through the modality of sign languages, such as the combination of vision and systematic gestures. It is essential that language be understood as the broader term that *includes* speech and sign language, because many people confuse speech and language with each other—a misunderstanding that has been the source of much unintended difficulty for deaf people.

9. *Language does not necessarily have a written form.* The written form is not a necessary characteristic; the majority of languages do not have one.

WHAT IS MEANT BY GRAMMAR?

Grammar, or the structure of language, consists of 1) *phonology* (how, in a spoken language, sounds go together to form words, or how, in a signed language, the elements of position, shape, and movement combine to form signs); 2) *syntax* (how words or signs are organized in sentences); 3) *semantics* (how to interpret the meaning of words, signs, and sentences); and 4) *pragmatics* (how to participate in a conversation, take turns, and anticipate the information needed by the person with whom you are communicating). Long before they start school, hearing children construct a grammar for their language that is eventually almost identical with that of all the other speakers of that language. They can then create and understand an unlimited number of sentences that they have never encountered before. They will know what is acceptable (and what is not) within their language system—a truly amazing feat.

In an excellent summary of the subject of language acquisition, Moskowitz (1978) points out that we tend to associate the word "grammar" with the rules of so-called correct usage that we were taught (and probably found boring) in grammar school. These rules, she states, are merely "the arbitrary finishing touches of embroidery on a thick fabric of language that each child weaves for herself before arriving in the . . . classroom. The fabric is grammar: the set of rules that describe how to structure language" (p. 92).

WHAT ARE THE EARLIEST ROOTS OF COMMUNICATION?

Many language researchers believe that the human brain has a built-in predisposition to acquire language. During the first year of life, infants and their mothers establish a communication system. Babies use eye gaze, body posture, head position, facial expression, and gestures in increasingly elaborate ways as dependable cues to inner emotional states. Caregivers learn to recognize whether infants are hungry, ready to be fed more, and so forth. This communication system is based largely on inborn automatic reflex mechanisms in the first few months of life, but later in the first year there is much more voluntary activity.

During their first year, infants can point and reach, make specific reference to something in the outside world, and often, at the same time, encode (show) their emotional attitude toward it. (The baby who does not like a particular food may not only struggle or push the hand offering it away, but may also make whining sounds and show a facial expression of disgust.) These patterns continue to be used in one form or another in later life as non-verbal communication, but are also important in cementing the relationship with the parents and in helping the child realize that experience has meaning. Thus, these patterns also assist in language development (Givens, 1978).

WHAT IS NON-VERBAL COMMUNICATION?

Hearing people use tone of voice, noises (such as sighs), shoulder shrugs, facial expressions, and gestures to accompany, to enrich, and to modify speech. Hearing people generally assume that this non-verbal communication is inferior to speech, because it seems to be more variable, less conscious, and not symbolic, systematic, or linguistic.

Obvious differences in non-verbal communication exist from one culture to another, but as yet not much is known about how this type of communication develops in children (Harper, Wiens, and Matarazzo, 1978; Mayo and La France, 1978).

A PROBLEM WITH DEFINITIONS

Whatever the differences between the sign and spoken languages, both modalities are systematic, specific, and symbolic (capable of communicating abstract ideas, such as "love," "many," and "later"). In this sense, languages in either modality are *verbal*. (Unfortunately, "verbal" is a confusing word because it is commonly used to mean "expressive" or "articulate.")

Non-verbal communication is often judged to be less important (second-class) in the communication of content, even though it would be difficult to do without this addition to our language. If sign languages are classed as a kind of non-verbal communication, they too will be regarded as second-class, inadequate systems, or, as has sometimes been stated, "a loose collection of gestures." The reason that sign languages have so often been misclassified as non-verbal systems of communication is probably because their form is visual-gestural, which is also the most common form of non-verbal communication for hearing people.

In fact, deaf people use non-verbal communication in much the same way that hearing people do. It is a relatively simple matter to separate speech from all the gestures and facial expressions that go with it. However, when deaf persons use both special and conventional gestures, body movement, and facial expression to replace the hearing person's intonations, most hearing people cannot distinguish the difference between the conventional gestures and the sign language that is occurring simultaneously.

It is important that you as a parent are aware of this sometimes mistaken classification: defining sign languages as non-verbal communication is not only wrong, but *danger-ous*. Deaf people deserve more consideration.

WHAT ARE THE STAGES OF LANGUAGE DEVELOPMENT?

It has been shown that by six weeks of age hearing children prefer the human voice to other sounds and can begin to distinguish among different voices. Gestures and eye contact with their parents are already a form of communication. By six months they are experimenting with their own voices (*babbling*). Around 12 months they make their first one-word utterances. (These may carry much more meaning than an adult's single word, especially when combined with non-verbal communication.)

At about 18 months of age two-word utterances appear. From this point on children rapidly expand their language toward the adult form. By age five this process is almost complete. Children do not merely imitate the adult language around them; in all the languages that have been studied, they have been found to follow a sequence of stages. Moores (1978b) has reviewed some of the processes thought to be involved in language development: 1) *imitation* of what adults say is important, but children may omit or change certain

parts of what they hear according to their level of grammatical development at the time (for example, "Mommy
go?"); 2) parents *expand* what their children say by feeding
back to them a more complete and adult form of the
utterance, perhaps helping children to test their understanding ("Yes, Mommy is going out for a while"); and 3) by
induction children unconsciously figure out for themselves
the grammatical rules that seem to apply to the language,
but in doing this they first overgeneralize. For example,
after children learn the "-ed" rule for the past tense of
English verbs, they may start to say "goed" for "went," and
"gotted" for "got." (This is not from imitation, because these
are not forms they have heard from adults.)

Although putting words together occurs around 18
months of age, exposure to language is present from birth.
Comprehension precedes expression; children have a great
deal of knowledge before they learn to express it. Unlike
deaf babies, hearing babies have had vast experience listening
to models of clear speech before they themselves speak.

It is important to realize that children acquire language
through *informal* exposure and through active use, not
through being taught the language. The home experience
is fundamental; parents function not as language teachers,
but as facilitators who enable their child to absorb the culture
and to make active use of their curiosity. Children use
language to express feelings, to make their parents laugh,
to postpone undesired events ("Can I stay up for five more
minutes?"), to evade telling the truth ("Maybe I did eat the
cookies—I can't remember"), and so on.

Many investigators of child language believe that there
is a "sensitive period" when a first language is acquired most
readily and rapidly; afterwards, learning becomes much
more difficult (Moores, 1978b). When does this "sensitive
period" end? Perhaps at age four to five, but researchers are
still uncertain, and there are probably individual differences
as well.

By the time children are five, they can communicate
about the past and future, can use fantasy, and can ask

when, how, and why things happen. Language is also important for internal use in thought, though not all thinking is in language. Actually, we know relatively little about language and thinking. Sometimes people are curious about how a deaf native signer thinks—is it in signs? Signs seem to be one way, but pictures, written language, and words of the spoken language (if there is enough hearing) may also be involved (Conrad, 1979).

[Philip Dale's book (1976) is a good source of general information about the stages of language development.]

HOW DOES LANGUAGE DEVELOPMENT DIFFER IN THE DEAF CHILD?

If the deaf child has deaf parents who use sign language from the time of the child's birth, language development in sign language will follow essentially the same course as speech development in hearing children (Bonvillian, Nelson, and Charrow, 1976). The babbling observed in hearing children also occurs in deaf children, but often decreases and disappears because they do not hear their own voices. Maestas y Moores (1980) videotaped seven deaf infants (who had deaf parents) in their homes. Their communications were relaxed and effective. By 16 months of age they were asking questions, combining language elements in normal ways, and using some fingerspelling.

Most deaf children have hearing parents who do not know for some time that their child is deaf (the average age of diagnosis is 20 months according to the study of Freeman, et al., 1975). For these children, early unplanned exposure to people talking has provided little or nothing in the way of language development. At age two or three, therefore, the average deaf child is not ready to concentrate on developing meaning and content, as can the hearing child or the deaf child with deaf parents. As Moores has stated:

They (deaf children of hearing parents) must try to filter meaning from English messages through inadequately developed phonological and grammatical systems. The result is frequently a distortion of the original message. The situation produces children . . . whose achievements are limited because of a failure to provide them with the basic tools of standard English grammar. [1978b, p. 115]

For the deaf child in most hearing families, there are risks of serious early language deprivation and of an inability to learn what is going on around them and why (*incidental learning*). The early emotional bond with the parents may also be more difficult to establish and to maintain.

This is not to say that deaf children without a formal sign language communicate nothing. In spite of adverse conditions, human infants have a strong desire to communicate, and it is well known that deaf babies can spontaneously develop their own simple sign system (Goldin-Meadow and Feldman, 1975).

Anyone who has worked with deaf children knows how often they lack basic explanations when these are needed. The Spradleys, for instance, described their feelings when four-year-old Lynn was seriously ill with meningitis: "Right now, when we needed to communicate with her the most, we could not. Our own daughter—and we hardly knew her! What if she never recovered?" (1978, p. 189).

An even more dramatic example was given by D. Dale (1974), from his experiences in an oral-only residential school:

> . . . in discussing school entry with a group of 10 deaf boys and girls, aged 15 years, in New Zealand, I was astonished to learn that in every case, when they first came into residence at the age of 5 or 6, they believed that they would never return to their homes again. One Maori boy, who had helped his father round up sheep and put them on a train to be slaughtered, even believed that when he was placed on a train with a group of other children, he was going to be killed himself. He said that the sight of his mother on the platform and some of the children in the train crying, as well as his father looking very upset, convinced him that this must be so. [p. 195]

It is worth noting that D. Dale is an oralist, and that although he gives us this chilling (and perhaps exaggerated) tale, he does not suggest that the provision of another system of dependable early communication would have been worth considering. With the use of sign language, this child's disturbing experience might have been avoided.

CONCLUSIONS

Early language development has tremendous implications for hearing parents of deaf children. Ways of eliminating or minimizing the problems of deaf children are considered later in this book.

Although deaf parents have advantages in raising a deaf child, hearing parents can also learn to communicate with their deaf child freely. The satisfaction that parents can have when early communication succeeds is well illustrated by an anecdote from one of the families in our early intervention program. A two and one-half-year-old deaf child had observed her parents signing grace at the dinner table: "Thank you, Jesus, for this food." One evening they saw her add (in sign language): ". . . and birds and candy."

SUMMARY

1. For deaf children of hearing parents who cannot
    sign, early oral-only communication is very
    frustrating. Sign language is another available
    modality for expressing language.
2. Recent research on language development
    indicates that children normally go through
    predictable stages of development, no matter
    what language they are learning.
3. Language is one kind of communication. It is
    systematic, symbolic, social, learned, variable,
    and evolving; it has a grammar or structure; and
    it can take a number of expressive or receptive
    forms.
4. Grammar of a spoken language may be said to
    consist of phonology (sounds), syntax (relation of
    words to each other), semantics (meaning), and
    pragmatics (how to socially structure a
    conversation). Sign languages have equivalent
    organization.
5. In the first year of a child's life, infants and their
    parents develop the roots of communication, even
    before the first words are used.
6. Hearing infants play with sounds (babble) at
    around six months of age. By age 12 months they
    utter their first words, and around age 18 months
    they start to combine words. By age four or five,
    having passed through what some believe is a
    "sensitive," or optimal period of easiest language
    learning, they are already sophisticated (although
    not perfect) users of the language of their culture.
    They know the structure of their language and
    can concentrate on expanding the content by
    actively using language to understand and to
    change their world. This amazing
    accomplishment is largely an outgrowth of
    informal experience.
7. Deaf infants in deaf families follow almost the
    same steps in language development, although

their babbling decreases and usually stops after about six months.

8. Non-verbal communication enriches verbal or symbolic communication, but is usually regarded as less important for conveying content. For this reason, it is essential not to define sign languages as non-verbal forms of communication. Sign languages are non-speech (some say non-oral), not non-verbal. Language does not equal speech.

9. Deaf children of hearing parents run serious risks of impeded development if they have no clear communication system. The problems may include a weakened emotional bond with parents and the lack of a dependable language system for thinking and incidental learning during the most important years. In addition, life experiences may become more than usually upsetting because the deaf child cannot get adequate explanations for why things happen.

Chapter 10

SPEECH, SPEECHREADING, AND AUDITORY TRAINING

Sign language is the hallmark of the deaf adult community. In reaction against the stigma placed upon their language, many deaf adults depreciate the value or even the usefulness of hearing aids, speech, or lipreading skills. [Schlesinger and Meadow, 1972, p. 3]

INTRODUCTION

In most books on hearing impairment, issues concerning hearing aids and auditory training are not treated as controversial, but we believe that they are. Our interest is not in the mechanics of various pieces of equipment or in the technical aspects of training procedures, but in several still unresolved issues, such as the lack of basic knowledge about how language develops.

In this chapter, we mention some generally accepted facts and methods concerning speech, speechreading, and auditory training and list some still unsettled questions. We delay giving any suggestions for solutions until Chapter 12, where we can put them into a Total Communication perspective. [More information, from an oralist perspective, is available from the A. G. Bell Association for the Deaf.]

Any parent whose child has used a hearing aid knows that there can be great frustration in getting the child to use it properly and in keeping it in serviceable condition.

Different professionals may make different or even contradictory statements or recommendations about the development of speech and speechreading skills. We have decided not to present the details of the many kinds of equipment used and of the ways of maintaining and using hearing aids; this information is constantly changing and is usually made available to parents when they purchase a hearing aid for their child. Information can also be easily obtained through schools, clinics, audiologists, and professional and parent organizations. [Two good sources are the booklets by Craig, Sins, and Rossi (1976a, 1976b), one for parents, the other for deaf children. More technical discussions may be found in Bess (1977) and Ross and Giolas (1978).]

In this chapter, we prefer to emphasize those aspects of expressive and receptive speech training that are not so readily available, especially to parents. In addition, we apply to our discussion the concept of differences among deaf children (both individual differences and those related to severity of hearing loss and age at onset of deafness).

SOME GENERALLY ACCEPTED FACTS

Most deaf children have some residual (remaining) hearing. The brain, which develops rapidly in the first few years of life, needs rich language input during that time. This is sometimes called a "sensitive," or optimal time for language development: thinking, emotional ties to the parents, and language should develop together (Furth, 1966). The concept of an optimal period does not mean that language cannot develop later, only that later it may be more difficult or may be separated from other important areas of development.

Parents and teachers become accustomed to listening to the speech of deaf children and, as a result, may judge it to be more useful in everyday life than it really is. In other words, we must distinguish between speech that is intelligible to strangers and speech that is intelligible only to those who know it well or only to those who know it in routine situations familiar to the child. Speechreading must be similarly judged. (The term "speechreading" is preferred to the more commonly used "lipreading" because it is not only the *lip* movements that are read.)

Conrad's extensive study (1979) of British deaf children at the end of their school careers showed that, when judged by strangers (or even by their own teachers), most had very poor speech. In spite of training, the average speechreading ability of those deaf teenagers was at best equal to that of untrained hearing teenagers of the same age.

Language is the key to speechreading, just as it is the key to reading. We do not break down words (read, spoken, or signed) into each of their smallest parts before understanding them. Instead, we anticipate *patterns* from what has gone before and from context. Even under the best of conditions, hearing people do not hear everything in speech, nor read everything in what they read. Most of the time this is unnecessary because there is a built-in redundancy (extra clues) in our language. Knowledge of the language must be available, however, in order for deaf children to give meaning to the even more limited input received from hearing and vision.

SOME UNSETTLED ISSUES

Because amplification only makes sounds louder (including the sounds distorted by sensory-neural deafness), there is question whether the abnormal amplified sound received by deaf children can be the basis for a "native" or first language. If the answer is yes, will this language be gained early enough to be usable when the developing child needs it most? If not, then the language of the surrounding majority must be acquired through a different channel (vision) or taught as a second language (Stevens, 1976).

If there is a sensitive, or best period in early life for language learning, through what techniques can this best be developed—auditory, oral (speechreading), signing, or a combination of some or all of these? Does the mode (auditory or visual) matter? Can several types of input be successfully received and integrated by the brain at the same time?

How long should one continue with a method of training without satisfactory results before giving up? Should one try again later if there is no success? What is the effect on a child of concentrating on what he or she cannot do well?

We simply do not have sufficient knowledge to answer all these questions as well as we would like. An argument can therefore be made for allowing the child's abilities to determine the decision, rather than restricting ourselves to a few possibilities, as if we already had the answers for all deaf children (Conrad, 1980).

HEARING AIDS

Purpose

The purpose of all amplification is to make the most of residual hearing, so that meaning can be attached to what is heard (even if only loud noises, and not speech, can be understood).

Features of Hearing Aids

All hearing aids have certain common features: a *microphone* (to convert sound into an electronic signal), an *amplifier* (to strengthen the signal), a loudspeaker or *earphone* (to convert the signal back into louder sound), a *power source* or battery, and a *volume* or *gain control*. Some hearing aids have tone controls allowing for emphasis or de-emphasis upon certain parts of the amplified sound range. Output controls set the upper limit of amplified sound that can be delivered. There may be a telephone attachment. Some aids have other features, such as directionality or an arrangement for receiving the teacher's voice via an FM receiver (Ross, 1977).

Earmolds

An individually fitted *earmold* fits snugly into the ear's external canal. If too much sound leaks around a loose mold, the microphone will pick it up and a feedback cycle will be started. This results in a squeal that is not helpful to the deaf child and is unpleasant for the hearing persons around the child. As the child grows, new earmolds must be fitted to maintain the snug fit.

Body Aids

From the beginning of this century until about 25 years ago, *body aids* were the only type of hearing aid available. They were worn on a harness around the neck, pinned to clothing, or secured in a pocket. A Y-cord divided the output to earphones for both ears. Separate binaural outputs to each ear are now available, or two separate body aids may be worn.

Body aids have several advantages, and are still used for very young deaf children and some older profoundly deaf children. The electronic components are larger, giving greater flexibility of design and greater durability and sturdiness (young children are very hard on such equipment); the batteries are larger, with longer life; and, because the microphone and earphones are further apart, there is less feedback or squeal. Body aids are generally capable of producing higher levels of output over a wider range than the ear-level aids. There are also some disadvantages: they are cumbersome and more visible (unsightly to some parents and deaf youth); when they are worn in a pocket or under a sweater, too much clothing noise is picked up; and their output is not as accurately binaural as ear-level aids because their microphones are not at ear level.

Ear-Level Aids

Ear-level aids are now used by the majority of hearing-impaired children. These are the type with all of the components behind the ear. (There are a few other variations not often used for children: aids built into eyeglasses or aids placed within the external ear.) The advantages of ear-level aids are greater acceptability (because they are less visible), and less clothing noise. New developments have made these aids almost as powerful as body aids. Their disadvantages are: shorter battery life, less durability, the need for precise earmold fit to prevent feedback, and somewhat more sound distortion.

Maintenance of Hearing Aids

Cost and maintenance are significant factors in acquiring and using an appropriate hearing aid. Small children tend to treat their aids very roughly, and servicing may not be immediately available. Unless a temporary replacement is provided, the deaf child may be without the hearing aid for days, weeks, or even longer, and this may happen repeatedly. Studies have shown that the hearing aids of many deaf children are not in working condition much of the time; the most common cause is dead batteries (Porter, 1973; Zink, 1972).

Early or Late Start for Amplification?

Although an early start for amplification is almost always assumed to be necessary, a recent Scandinavian study (Nordén, 1980) described good results from the use of amplification that was begun late. The children, who were in a Total Communication program, had good language development and had already started to read. Further research is needed on this issue, however.

WHY SOME DEAF CHILDREN DO NOT USE THEIR AIDS

> Three-year-old Mark refused to wear his hearing aid. Although his teacher kept emphasizing the need for him to use it during his waking hours, this advice was difficult for his parents to follow, because he kept pulling it out and fussed when it was replaced. Much effort went into distracting him so that, without removing it frequently, he gradually got used to how it felt.
>
> I have seen parents who force the hearing aid to a point of driving the child crazy. It can become an obsession to parents if they do not look at it from the child's point of view. [Quote from a parent]

There are several common, well-recognized reasons for resistance to wearing hearing aids: the earmold may not fit well and can irritate the ear; a skin irritation of the external canal may make the earmold painful to wear; the aid may not suit the child's hearing loss; or the volume may be set too high, especially when recruitment occurs (as described in Chapter 4). Of course, it is also possible that the child simply has too little hearing for amplification to be of any use.

There are also parental attitudes to contend with. Despite the fact that hearing aids have been greatly improved in recent years, the aid may not live up to parental expectations or hopes, which may have been unrealistic. Wearing a hearing aid may be embarrassing because it calls attention to the fact that the deaf child is different. The aid may also cost too much to keep in repair, and it may seem unfair to force the child to wear it. Some deaf parents of deaf children may not have found their own hearing aids to be of much (or any) help, or their own education may have created negative attitudes toward hearing aids and auditory training. These feelings could cause a biased attitude toward their own child's training. Deaf children can pick up these attitudes and resist even more strongly because of them.

Older children may become aware that they are different from others and may resent this fact; the hearing aid can be symbolic of this difference. The child or parents may also feel bad about the emphasis upon what the child *cannot* do: hear normally.

Children differ in the ease with which they adjust to new situations (such as wearing an aid), both from child to child and from age to age in their individual development. Some otherwise normal children are difficult for their parents to manage because they have certain behavior patterns: being highly persistent, having intense reactions, and/or displaying a frequently negative mood. It may be hard work to encourage such children to use a new piece of equipment that they must feel next to their body and must accept as part of themselves. At ages two or three many children are normally rather stubborn and oppositional (the so-called terrible twos), and they are not yet easy to influence through persuasion.

For the degree of deafness we are considering in this book, improved responses through aided hearing (when they come about at all) are likely to be only slowly developed and will not reward child or parent as quickly as the immediate positive two-way communication of sign language. (This issue is discussed in greater detail in Chapter 12.)

When resistance is encountered, parents who believe that the use of an aid is important will have to examine several elements (probably with the assistance of the child's teacher, audiologist, or otologist): the hearing aid itself (earmold and adjustment); their own attitudes; and the child's overall needs, areas of strength and weakness, developing attitudes toward deafness, and experiences with other children. Once identified, the "costs" of solving the problem may need to be weighed against the benefits.

AUDITORY TRAINING

Most people seem to think that if they—deaf persons—have got a hearing aid they should be normal. You know—"If they've got a hearing aid why can't they hear you, why can't they come out and speak." They just don't understand. It's the general feeling that if you've got a hearing aid it's like some magic box that puts everything right. [A mother from Gregory's study, 1976, p. 197]

Indeed, the use of a hearing aid is *not* like acquiring "a magic box." Nor is it at all like correcting common visual problems with eyeglasses. For a deaf child to benefit from amplification (if this is, in fact, possible), it will take time and effort. Even if amplification is useful for communicating with one person in quiet circumstances, it may be of little or no use in a group and/or in noisy situations.

Sometimes the teacher of the deaf child and the parents may use auditory (or speech) training equipment. The general advantages of such equipment over a hearing aid alone have been summarized by Rubin (1979): 1) better quality sound with less distortion; 2) a constant level of input even when the child moves far away from the sound source; 3) better control of environmental noise in relation to the teacher's voice; 4) wider range of individual adjustment of the equipment; and 5) lower cost over time, with greater ease of repair and maintenance.

There are several different types of auditory training equipment. In the past, *hard-wire systems* were used; these required all components to be directly hooked up to each other. Then an *induction loop* system was developed: the amplified signal is fed into a wire or loop that goes around the classroom and the telephone pick-up coils in the children's hearing aids pick up this signal. If more than one classroom is using such a system, there can be *spillover* of the electrical field, causing interference. A modification using an FM broadcasting device is now available and is suitable for some children. Both children and teacher can move around, and there is no spillover because each room uses a different frequency, as radio stations do.

SPEECH TRAINING FOR DEAF CHILDREN

Speech Intelligibility

At present the majority of deaf children do not develop intelligible speech (Conrad, 1979), and there seems to be no dependable way to predict which of them will: ". . . children who have residual hearing and who present similar audi-

ograms may show very different speech reception abilities"
(Stark, 1979, p. 232).

Usefulness of Speech

This does not mean that speech is of no use, either receptively
(hearing or speechreading) or expressively (talking). Most
deaf adults value whatever speech or speechreading skills
they possess, as this description by one of our deaf resource
people illustrates:

> My wife was born profoundly deaf and to most strangers her speech is hard to
> understand. An example is the time when she started her first job in a large office.
> On the first day only one girl had some idea of what Anne said, so she had to
> write everything down (she has good language), but after a few months practically
> all of her workmates had got used to her pronunciation. Thereafter she rarely had
> to write anything down. My experience as a social worker has also shown that
> hearing people closely associated with prelingually deaf people can often un-
> derstand their speech. The tragedy for most born-deaf people is that their reading
> and writing level is so low that they have little to talk about. A better education
> would enhance their oral ability, especially with close friends and workmates—
> there would be much more to talk about! Total Communication will certainly
> improve the all-round knowledge of deaf people, because the deaf children of
> deaf parents have proved this point. [Davis, personal communication, 1980]

In spite of whatever efforts deaf persons make, ". . . some
three-quarters have speech of little use for ordinary communication . . . There can be no escape from the conclusion
that speech communication between hearing and profoundly
deaf people remains a problem of immense magnitude"
(Conrad, 1979, p. 216).

Deaf Speech

The production and comprehension of speech sounds is
very complicated and still poorly understood (Ross and
Giolas, 1978). How does deaf speech differ from normal
speech? There are many descriptions, but almost none of
the identified characteristics adequately describe *all* deaf
children's speech. In general, the rate tends to be slower.
Timing, rhythm, and intonation are abnormal; breath, loud-

ness, and pitch control are unusual. Syllables may be added or omitted, and the tongue may not be properly placed to make some consonant sounds, especially those that cannot be observed on the lips.

Good sound production requires good receptive skills, usually through hearing, or perhaps via some supplementary means. There are various electronic sensory aids that have been used, such as vibrators and simplified visual displays of sounds. (The idea is an old one, and is reported to have been used by Alexander Graham Bell in 1874.) Although they are interesting, these and newer research techniques have not yet solved the problem of making deaf people perceive enough speech *as it is happening* to aid in their own speech development. As Conrad (1979) points out, the speech model that deaf children have available to them is defective because of their hearing loss. They must use this model and whatever they can remember of the feelings (from their own efforts to speak) in throat, jaw, lips, and tongue. This is a formidable task. There are limits to how much usable speech can be achieved under these circumstances. Perhaps more children with speech potential will be helped to reach their best level of speech comprehension and production, but only poor or fair speech intelligibility can be expected for most.

Speech Intelligibility and Internal Speech

Conrad (1979) claims that deaf children need a creative, freely usable language for *internal speech* (the practice of talking to ourselves, as most of us do when we are thinking). Conrad's research shows that if vocal speech is not intelligible (at least to parents), it does not function well for thinking. In other words, the idea that a deaf child who cannot sign and who has very poor speech is at least doing well in thinking is probably not correct. The nature of thought in relation to language is far from clear, however.

General Acceptance of Amplification

Most teachers of the deaf support the use of residual hearing through the use of hearing aids and auditory training. An awareness of the rhythm of speech, even if words themselves cannot be heard, may assist in speechreading once sufficient vocabulary is known. Ling (1978), for example, prefers the use of meaningful speech in auditory training, feeling that not much is accomplished by using noisemakers.

Controversies About Auditory or Visual Emphasis

There are few, if any, professionals who would argue that useful hearing should be ignored, but there are strong differences of opinion among the oralists over a number of issues. The controversy should not be surprising, but it is often not made clear to parents, who may believe that advice is based upon solid scientific evidence (when it is, in fact, lacking), or who may think that the only controversy is the so-called oral-manual one. A major issue is the emphasis on, and timing of, visual training (speechreading or cued speech) in relationship to auditory training. Those who favor an *acoupedic* (also known as "unisensory," "auditory," or "aural") approach believe in the training of hearing and *not* of vision (speechreading) in the early stages. Using the visual channel, it is feared, will make the child too dependent upon vision instead of the auditory channel (Ling, 1978). Others believe the reverse—that hearing should be a supplement to speechreading.

Individual versus Group Aids

The question whether children should wear their ear-level individual aids all day or whether they should use hard-wire, loop, or radio types of group equipment in school is also unsettled. Some teachers believe that two different auditory inputs will confuse the deaf child, but the evidence for this is unclear (Ross and Giolas, 1978, p. 319). At the moment the only answer seems to be to individualize decisions and to depend upon the best clinical judgment that is available.

Cued Speech

At Gallaudet College, Cornett (1967) has developed a system called *cued speech*. Twelve different hand shapes and positions are used around the face while speaking. In combination with certain sounds, these hand signals make it possible to better distinguish those speech sounds that are easily confused because they look the same on the lips. Cued speech is a tool, not a method in itself. It is *not* a language, and has no relationship to any type of sign language. Accepted by some oralists and not by others, it is perhaps most often considered a prop to aid speechreading. (An older, similar system, still in use, is Forchhammer's mouth-hand system in Denmark.)

Interest in cued speech has waxed and waned in several countries (U.S.A., Canada, Australia, the U.K.), but at no time has it been used with large numbers of deaf children. How effective is it? A two-year follow-up study by Clarke and Ling (1976) showed modest benefit. Recently a much more elaborate study was performed by Nicholls (1979) in Australia. She studied 19 prelingually profoundly deaf children who had been in a cued speech program for at least four years. The age of starting the program ranged from two through nine years. To summarize the findings briefly, all children did much better on word recognition tests through speechreading and cueing together than through speechreading alone. On the average, the results were not different with amplification added. Speechreading in situations where cues were unavailable did not seem to be adversely affected. This interesting study seems worthy of note. The authors admit, however, that it does not answer several questions: How early can cued speech be used in an early intervention program with very young deaf children? What will the long-term effects be? How do these results compare with other approaches?

Other Techniques

The use of the analytic method (using grammatical "keys" to sentences) and of the natural method (encouraging children to learn and to use words in real-life situations) has a long history. Many teachers employ combinations of methods, including vibration, music, residual hearing, visual displays of speech, fingerspelling, and syllable drill. These techniques may make varying contributions to speech reception, speech discrimination, and speech production.

Speechreading

There is no well-established method for the teaching of speechreading (Farwell, 1976). Why is it so difficult a process for deaf children? The child trying to speechread must know the vocabulary and grammar of the language, because (in English) about half the sounds are not visually distinguishable on the lips. Therefore, the meaning of words must be extracted from clues provided by the situation and by the topic of discussion. In English, for example, *"bad," "pat,"* and *"mat"* may be easily confused with each other. The child who knows the language well may decode these words when they are used in a sentence, but still may not be able to distinguish "You're bad" from "You're mad" except by guessing from what happened previously. Children with postlingual onset of deafness will speechread better because they already have a good command of the spoken language. It should also be noted that many of the speechreading techniques used by teachers were originally developed for hard-of-hearing adults, who had little or no problem with language and speech.

The Need for Further Research

In a useful summary of training techniques, Moores (1978b) has criticized efforts to teach speech to deaf children as haphazard and poorly researched. The different methods have never been adequately evaluated in comparison with each other, nor are there good diagnostic tests to measure speech development in deaf children.

CONCLUSIONS

Summarizing the many techniques of auditory/oral training and the beliefs and assumptions on which they are based is not easy. It is best to evaluate any method only as part of a total program that meets the needs of individual deaf children. The development of better speech and speechreading in a child who already has a good command of at least one language (even if it is not the native one) is not the same as attempting to use these approaches to provide a deaf child with a first language or "mother tongue." Judgments about the relative worth of various training methods tend to be variable and seem to depend more upon personal values and experience than upon solid evidence.

Generally, a period of early amplification is considered to be desirable, although how early this needs to be started is not clear. "The earlier the better" is advice that is often taken for granted, but the value of an early start has not really been adequately demonstrated.

Ideal conditions are rarely achieved. Instead of questioning the wisdom of their restrictive approach, oralists may claim that the admittedly poor results of oral-only training are from not making the diagnosis early enough, not starting with amplification early enough, not having a correctly fitted aid, not having enough well-trained staff, not having motivated parents who insist upon consistent use of the aid, and not having the appropriate school placement, among other reasons (Conrad, 1979). Ling (1978) states that "current knowledge, diligently applied, can lead to the acquisition of *fluent* spoken language skills by *most* hearing-impaired children" (p. 210, emphasis added). Given the real conditions in the world today—the shortage of funds for adequate medical and other services and the competing needs within families—the conditions for success are ideals that some might wish to strive toward; but these conditions are also a ready excuse for what others regard as "failures" in the basic approach to the deaf child.

Some parents may expect (and have been promised) too much too soon, only to abandon hearing aids and auditory training later, even though there might be some benefit. Others (such as some deaf parents) may decide that the training effort is not worth it for very limited goals, or they may think that their own bad experience is a good predictor of what their child is likely to go through. Whatever plan is adopted, consideration should be given to the possible negative effects upon the deaf child's self-image of practicing the very thing that he or she cannot do.

Auditory training devices, integrated with the child's hearing aid or independent of it, may be used by some parents and in some schools. The benefits must be evaluated over time.

A question that was raised earlier has yet to be addressed: Can several different types of auditory and visual input, if presented simultaneously, be integrated and used by the brain? Although Ling (1978) doubts that this is possible, it seems clear to us that it is (Meadow, 1980; see also Chapter 12).

What happens to those children who fail to develop language quickly enough when auditory/oral techniques are their sole source of input? Ling and Ling (1978) recommend switching to a Total Communication program if sufficient gains are not made by a deaf child in an oral-only program within 18–24 months. (This is still an unfortunately long delay, and quite unnecessary. Many oral programs keep children much longer than this, confronting parents with the reality of hindered development at school-entering age or even later.)

The teaching of speech articulation and speechreading is not in itself controversial. Instead, the emphasis that should be given to these communication skills relative to the other communicative and developmental needs of the deaf child arouses much debate.

There are many unsettled issues in this field that demand better research and follow-up. It would be truly beneficial for deaf children and for their families if professionals and organizations could cooperate in designing and carrying out needed research projects that could clarify many of the obscure areas touched upon in this chapter.

SUMMARY

1. A distinction must be made between techniques that try to *improve* a deaf child's speech and speechreading skills, based upon existing language, and restrictive methods that aim to develop a native language solely through auditory/oral means. The method for improvement is generally accepted, while the more restrictive method is highly controversial.

2. It is generally agreed that the best age for introducing amplification is as early as possible. (There is some recent evidence that it may be just as good, or better, to wait until the child is older, understands what is desired, and has more language and better motivation, but this theory needs further research.) The decision about when to start training depends partly upon one's belief in a "sensitive period" for sound and language input to the brain, and upon one's choice of the channel(s) of communication likely to be most useful for the child.

3. Hearing aids have several common features: a microphone, an amplifier, a battery, and an earphone. Usually the sound is directed into the external ear through an individually fitted earmold. Body aids are still useful for very young children; older children often use ear-level aids. (Each style of hearing aid has its own unique advantages and limitations.)

4. The use of a hearing aid does not mean that the child can easily make good use of residual hearing or can distinguish the sounds of speech. The capacity to use limited and distorted sounds for speech development, if present, must be patiently trained. Some children, even with the best and most consistently used aids, cannot hear speech (especially in less than ideal situations), although awareness both of noises and of the rhythm of speech may be useful.

5. Some deaf children resist using their hearing aids. Possible reasons include uncomfortable

earmolds, poorly adjusted amplification, lack of sufficient hearing for amplification to be useful, parent and child attitudes, and lack of significant help from amplification.

6. Auditory training equipment is available that makes it possible to deliver constant sound levels to each child in a classroom while limiting environmental noise. Both the teacher and the children are free to move about the classroom.

7. The speech of most deaf children and adults is presently very poor in spite of training. There is often abnormality in rhythm, breathing, rate, pitch, and volume. Their speechreading ability is also likely to be poor. Training in these skills has not been based upon good research.

8. There are a wide variety of receptive and expressive speech training techniques used by different schools and teachers. None seems very successful with most *deaf* children, although individual successes may be demonstrated with any method. It is therefore impossible to give firm general recommendations.

9. Cued speech has shown some promise in improving speechreading in profoundly deaf children. Further research is necessary to determine whether it can provide a means of learning a native spoken language.

10. Deaf adults often report that their speech skills, although limited, are of considerable use to them.

11. Parents sometimes have unrealistically high expectations of hearing aids and auditory training. Although these aids often *are* of value, there may be serious disappointment if excellent speech and speechreading are the expected result.

12. As long as the goal of early enjoyable *language interchange* is not forgotten, attempts to develop useful speech and speechreading seem reasonable.

Chapter 11

SIGN LANGUAGES
Myth and Reality

. . . Oh, better
The word in hand than a thousand
spilled from the mouth upon the
hearless ear. [Dorothy Miles (1976)]

Oh I don't mind gesture. I think if they can understand anything it's better than
not understanding at all . . .

. . . Well we can't really stop him because it's the only means of communication
with him—see if we stopped that and relied on his voice we wouldn't get nowhere
with him. We've got to use signs to him, though we do try and make him so he
doesn't use the signs. [Two English mothers quoted in Gregory, 1976, pp.
126–127]

INTRODUCTION

These three selections show how varied the feelings about
sign language can be: the pride and confidence of a deaf
poet; the recognition of the necessity to use signs (but with
a hint that this is second-class) by one mother; and the
apologetic and clearly mixed feelings of another mother.
Few methods of communication have been subjected to
greater misunderstanding and repression than sign language. Parents have been made to fear it by some of their
advisers, deaf children have been punished for using it, its
use has been made illegal in some areas, and many of the
teachers and parents of the very same children who will
grow up to be signing deaf adults cannot communicate with
them in this mode or language.

Table 2.   A Sign Language Quiz

Statement	Response
	Yes No
1. Sign language is universal (deaf people from anywhere in the world can easily understand each other).	( ) ( )
2. Sign language is instinctive. It develops from primitive gestures that children make even without instruction or imitation.	( ) ( )
3. Sign languages are easier for hearing people to learn than spoken languages.	( ) ( )
4. Sign languages are ungrammatical.	( ) ( )
5. Sign languages are concrete (can only express ideas that can be pictured by the hands).	( ) ( )
6. Sign languages are much faster at transmitting information than spoken languages.	( ) ( )
7. Sign languages are much slower at transmitting information than spoken languages.	( ) ( )
8. Sign languages cannot convey subtle shades of meaning.	( ) ( )
9. The use of sign language by a deaf child will prevent speech development.	( ) ( )

Sign language is an emotionally loaded subject. Before reading further about sign languages and attitudes toward them, we suggest that you take the quiz found in Table 2.

The answer to all of the statements in Table 2 is no. Nevertheless, many people who should know better believe some or all of them.

The remainder of this chapter discusses sign languages and various "invented" sign codes or systems that are intended to represent spoken languages. Although there has been an explosion of knowledge in this previously neglected field, there is still much misunderstanding and confusion.

THE NATURE OF SIGNING

Introduction

Although signing can be a confusing subject, parents need some basic understanding of it. If you have chosen a Total

Communication program for your child, there may still be important questions to answer: What language should you use first with your deaf baby, before a school program begins? If you are advised to use a sign code, should it be supplemented with a native sign language, and if so, how? If your local school or educational authority has decided on a specific manually coded system, how can you be sure which one is best? What will the relationship of your child be, as a user of such a system, to members of the deaf community?

The many recent changes in understanding sign languages and sign codes bring with them the danger of replacing with new myths those that have been discredited. Some of these myths have been clearly identified by Caccamise (1978). We have no desire to see additional problems created, but all progress generates new questions and revisions of our present understanding will undoubtedly be needed as well.

Some Important Distinctions

Although some writers include both sign languages and sign codes under the general heading of manual communication, we prefer not to do so, because it wrongly suggests that only the *hands* are used linguistically. (There is also non-manual linguistic information.) We will refer to *sign languages* when we mean an independent language, and to a *sign code* when discussing an invented system that is used to code a spoken language.

Signing is developing so rapidly that confusing changes in terminology are bound to occur. Don't be discouraged! You will soon identify those issues that are important to understand. Fortunately, improved reading and teaching materials are being produced and will be much more readily available than in the past.

Cued Speech and Fingerspelling

Although *cued speech* makes use of the hands, it is basically a support for speechreading and is not a sign language.

Fingerspelling is not a language in itself, but a code for conveying the spelling of words, like Morse Code. It is a kind of "writing in the air," whether it be of English or of some other language. (Some writers point out, however, that when young children use fingerspelling, the hand movements become, in effect, a "sign" in themselves, just like reading a whole word rather than a series of letters.)

There are several fingerspelling systems. One-handed systems are used in North America, Scandinavia, and the Soviet Union, among other countries. Each letter has its own hand-shape. (In the United Kingdom, Australia, and parts of the British Commonwealth, a two-handed system is used.) When speech is used simultaneously with one-handed fingerspelling, it is known as the *Rochester Method* (Visible English) or *neo-oralism* in the Soviet Union.

There are several disadvantages to fingerspelling if used alone or used simultaneously with speech. First, you must know the language and its written form; it cannot be used as a first language because little children do not yet know the spelling of their parents' language and do not have sufficient eye/hand coordination. Also, it is slow, cannot approximate normal speech rhythm, and is less emotionally expressive. These limitations are discussed by Bornstein (1979a and 1979b), Caccamise, Hatfield, and Brewer (1978), and Wilbur (1979).

Nevertheless, fingerspelling is important. It is used for words that do not have sign language equivalents or that are not in the user's vocabulary. It is also used for proper names and may influence the development of new signs. [The educational uses and limitations of fingerspelling are discussed further in Chapter 18.]

What are Sign Languages?

Unlike fingerspelling or cued speech, sign languages are independent languages; they have their own structure and grammar and their own community of users (both native ones and those who learned it later). Signs are gestural-visual symbols that are used regularly and systematically. They are constructed from combinations of hand-shapes and movements of the hands and other parts of the body in relation to each other.

It has already been argued (in Chapter 9) that sign languages are not *non-verbal* forms of communication. They are *non-speech* or *non-oral*. In fact, one of the possible sources of confusion about sign languages is that deaf persons tend to be well practiced in pantomime. It is this facility that helps them to communicate with deaf users of foreign sign languages, but there is *no* universal sign language (Battison and Jordan, 1980).

Only about 10% of deaf children have deaf parents. Sign language for young deaf children with hearing parents has been strongly discouraged until recently. This has created a unique situation compared to other languages—most deaf children do not acquire a native sign language from their hearing parents, but from their deaf peers or from deaf adults. The use of a native sign language usually identifies a person as a member of the deaf community.

What is meant by a *native* language as applied to sign languages? Any language learned from birth (a "mother tongue") is native; those who acquired a full range of sign language capabilities in early life are usually considered *native signers*. Although it is sometimes said that sign language is the native or natural language of deaf people, that does not mean that all deaf persons learn one sign language automatically (any more than everyone who is hearing learns English). At the present time relatively few deaf people are native signers, but sign languages are the only naturally evolved languages that are capable of being acquired by deaf children in very early life in a way and at a rate comparable to the language acquisition of hearing children.

Most hearing parents of deaf children never learn a native sign language. If they do learn to sign, it is in a form closer to the spoken language.

The best studied of all of the sign languages is American Sign Language, also known as Ameslan, or simply ASL. ASL is also used, with variations, in most of Canada; French-Canadian Sign Language is used by many French-Canadian deaf persons; and derivatives of British Sign Language are in use in the Maritime Provinces. Many of these deaf Canadians are bilingual—using two sign languages. Many of the statements made about sign languages in this chapter apply specifically to ASL. The extent to which they apply to other sign languages must be determined by the results of continuing research.

The study of British Sign Language, or BSL, is only just beginning (Brennan and Colville, 1979; Deuchar, 1979). Other sign languages that are being studied include Australian (Power, personal communication, 1980), Israeli (Namir and Schlesinger, 1978), and Swedish (Bergman, 1978, 1979).

Structure and Grammar of Sign Languages

Code-switching. We all change our way of talking (and writing) depending upon the person, topic, or situation with which we are dealing. We do not talk to children or to those who do not speak our language well in the same way as we speak with our peers. This *code-switching* (as it is called by linguists) is evident in all languages, including sign languages (Preisler, 1980). Such changes are performed automatically. For example, we may change from the more formal language used in giving a speech to the more informal code used among our family and friends. (Baby-talk and "childrenese" are good examples of code-switching.)

Influence of spoken languages. Sign languages do not parallel the structure of spoken languages and are thus harder for hearing people to understand and to accept. As a result, sign languages have been subject to discrimination and to efforts to stamp them out (Lane, 1980). Sign languages are not usually taught in schools, where children are supposed to learn the majority language. Surrounding spoken languages have influenced sign languages, as they do any minority language. Culture, prestige, educational theories, and the need to communicate across the deaf/hearing linguistic boundary have all exerted pressures on the languages of deaf people. Consequently, there is a gradation (or *continuum*) between the native sign language and the form of signing that can represent the spoken language.

Pidgins or blends. When two languages have extensive contact with each other, a mixture of the two usually develops, called a *pidgin,* or *blend.* This has happened, for example, where trade has been extensive between English-speaking traders and peoples using African, Polynesian, and other languages. Pidgins are characterized by a mixture of the structures of two languages, by a simplification of grammar and vocabulary, and by use in restricted social situations. They are no one's *native* language. When people who are deaf communicate in signs with hearing people who are not native signers, they use as much of the spoken language structure as they know. Signing that is intermediate between the native sign language (such as ASL) and a manually coded English are usually referred to as Pidgin

Signing and Sign Languages

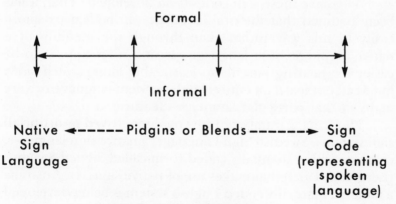

Figure 9. Signing and sign languages.

Sign English, or PSE (Woodward and Markowicz, 1980).
(The synonyms "siglish" or "Sign English" may also be
encountered.) An oversimplified diagram of this situation is
shown in Figure 9.

Pidgins are natural developments, not constructed language systems. In the case of PSE, ASL signs are strung
together in English word order along with some fingerspelling and the use of ASL features like directionality. Pidgin
sign languages have only been studied very recently; much
is still to be learned.

SYSTEMS OF SIGN (SIGN CODES)

The sign codes or systems currently in use are outgrowths
of the increasing acceptance of non-oral communication and
of the desire to teach deaf children the majority oral language
by manual means. Sign codes have been designed to convey,
insofar as possible, the detailed structure and grammar of
the spoken language. They are not independent languages.
(We stress that they have been invented *as a system,* whereas
native and pidgin sign languages have naturally evolved,
retaining those features that continue to be useful and
efficient.) Native sign languages may, however, adopt or
invent new signs.

Why have these sign codes been developed? First, it has
been assumed that the oral language can be learned more
easily in this way rather than through the medium of a
native or pidgin sign language. Second, they appear to be
easier for hearing parents to learn; they must switch *mode,*
but need not learn an entirely independent language or very
many of that particular language's features.

There are a number of invented (contrived or artificial)
sign systems. Swedish Sign Language, a native sign language,
co-exists with a manually coded form called Signed Swedish
(Bergman, 1979) that makes use of native signs. In Australia
a national manually coded English system is being developed
(Reynolds, personal communication, 1980).

In Britain there is a different and peculiar situation. A system was designed 30 years ago by Sir Richard Paget and developed further by Lady Grace Paget and Dr. Pierre Gorman, now known as the Paget-Gorman Sign System, or PGSS. Unfortunately PGSS seems to have been developed in almost total isolation from the language of the deaf community: the sign vocabulary of PGSS is not related to British Sign Language and is not intelligible to British deaf people. Children learning PGSS will have nothing linguistically in common with deaf adults, which is a distinct disadvantage.

The North American scene appears more complicated than it actually is in practice. At least five codes for English have been invented, but all take much of their sign vocabulary from ASL. Although this does not allow parents to understand ASL, it at least provides an entry point for productive contacts with deaf adults. Each of these codes attempts to duplicate the structure of English in different ways. [Good discussions of these codes can be found in Bornstein (1979a and 1979b) and Wilbur (1979).] These systems probably do not adhere quite as closely to English as their inventors might believe (Bornstein, 1979a; Charrow, 1976). They are presently undergoing revision and improvement. Seeing Essential English (SEE-1), Signing Exact English (SEE-2), Manual English, and Signed English are the codes now in use.

Please note that Signed English is not the same as the term sometimes used for PSE, "Sign English." Another confusion is caused by the term "Manual English," which is used in at least three ways in North America: 1) as a general term for all manually coded English systems; 2) as a synonym for fingerspelling and speech (Rochester Method or Visible English); and 3) as the modification of SEE-1 developed at the Washington State School for the Deaf. In Britain, manual English refers to an adaptation of British Sign Language to make it parallel English (Evans, 1979). Because of this possible confusion, clarification should be requested whenever someone refers to manual English.

The World Federation of the Deaf has also devised an international sign vocabulary called Gestuno (not an independent language) for use at international meetings (British Deaf Association, 1975).

The invented codes have sometimes aroused hostility and scorn from deaf adults. There are probably two major reasons for this opposition. First, their native sign languages have not been accorded sufficient dignity, and for years they have had to tolerate hearing experts on deafness, who try to tell them how to communicate. Second, certain linguistic distortions are created by these sign codes with which it is easy to find fault (Kannapell, 1978; Meadow, 1980). The process is inevitably a compromise—parts of one language that developed in a visual-gestural mode are being used to code another language adapted to a vocal-auditory mode. The systems generally try to have one sign stand for one word of the spoken language, which has sometimes created bad feelings. Deaf people may believe that this is part of an effort to ignore perfectly good native signs, and to stamp out their language and culture. For example, an English word for which there is one native sign may be broken down into a root (for which the sign code has chosen a different sign), plus other endings. For example, the word *gravy* might be signed "grave + y" or *accompany* might be signed "a + come + pan + y." Another example is the English word *right,* which has *three* signs in ASL representing the concepts of direction (to the *right*), correctness (that's *right*), and entitlement (I have a *right* to it). Kannapell (1978) has reviewed some of these linguistic and cultural objections of deaf people to manual codes.

Although we appreciate the strong feelings that language issues arouse, we feel that it is appropriate to look on the positive side of these efforts to develop a manually coded system, *provided* there is flexibility of application and a sincere appreciation of native sign languages. Research projects in the next few years are likely to tell us more about how various sign codes and sign languages can be utilized for the benefit of deaf children. Premature choice of one manual code for *all* deaf children, rejecting native and pidgin sign languages, would be not only unnecessary but also highly destructive.

There has already been some assimilation of invented signs into ASL, just as English has adopted words from many other languages. Deaf adults are not necessarily opposed to new signs. In practice there is some mutual intelligibility between the PSE used by deaf children or adults in conversing with hearing people and the invented codes learned by many teachers and parents.

THE STRUCTURE OF AMERICAN SIGN LANGUAGE

The linguistic study of native sign languages is very recent. The remarks that follow pertain to ASL. Results of close study have overturned most or all of the previously held ideas about this language.

If you are interested in more details than we can provide here, two excellent non-technical booklets are available, one by Markowicz (1977) and the other by Baker and Padden (1978a). Hoemann (1979) has presented a brief and readable account of much recent research, and has provided teaching materials as well (1975). The books by Klima and Bellugi (1979) and Wilbur (1979) cover all aspects of ASL (in rather technical language). William Stokoe of Gallaudet College's Linguistic Research Laboratory was the first to study ASL linguistically. His earlier works have been re-published in revised form (Stokoe, 1978; Stokoe, Casterline, and Croneberg, 1976). Stokoe also publishes a journal on all aspects of sign languages (*Sign Language Studies*) and a newsletter, *Signs for Our Times*. Other recent books are by Baker and Battison (1980, highly recommended). Battison (1978), Friedman (1977), Liben (1978), Royal National Institute for the Deaf (1976), Schlesinger and Namir (1978), and Siple (1978). There are also several relevant articles in previous issues of the *American Annals of the Deaf* subsequent to the early 1970s.

At the end of this book we have provided much more than our usual references and suggested reading list for this subject, because the results of recent work are as yet unknown to many parents and professional workers. Books for learning ASL and sign vocabulary are coming out so quickly that no full list can be given here. O'Rourke (1978) is a popular reference for vocabulary, and a new ASL series should also be helpful (Cokely and Baker, in press). A work on BSL has just been published (Brennan et al., 1980).

We can summarize from the study of ASL the following elements: sign languages use space and time by the actions of the hands, face, eyes, head, and other parts of the body to perform some of the grammatical functions that in spoken (oral) languages are done by volume, tone of voice, intonation, special words, word order, word endings, or modifications within words (*inflections*, such as man/men, go/goes) (Baker and Padden, 1978b). Much of this information about the structure of ASL was missed by those who wrote about sign languages before ASL was studied as a language.

The basic isolated form of a sign, such as is pictured in most sign language books, is known as a *citation* form. Putting together a string of citation-form signs is no more like ASL than trying to create French by inserting French words into their dictionary-equivalent slots in an English sentence. Sometimes sign language sentences are transposed into a written form in English (*glossed*) as if nothing more were being communicated than a string of citation-form signs made with the hands. This telegraphic form of English may then be criticized as a primitive or inadequate kind of communication. Such "translations" definitely do not convey all of the information that the signing does.

In addition to non-manual information, changes are also imposed on the citation form of the signs (just as they are on the pronunciation of isolated words when they are used in sentences). As linguists put it, there are *constraints* on the formation of signs. What is recognized as grammatical or acceptable in one sign language may not be in another. Slips of the hand, like slips of the lip or tongue, show that the mistakes made are not random, but are rather systematic within any one sign language (Klima and Bellugi, 1979).

Criticisms made of ASL in the past have usually been based upon misunderstandings. For example, it was wrongly claimed that all ASL signs bear a direct pictorial relationship to what is meant, technically known as *iconicity*. (The sign for "milk" is an opening and closing of both hands as if milking a cow. Some signs may be remembered by hearing learners because the sign looks like what is being described, but few signs have obvious meanings to the person who does not know sign language. Claims of iconicity imply that sign languages cannot express abstract meanings that cannot be pictured. Although it makes more use of mime in the origin of some signs, ASL is not limited to this possibility. If it were, you could expect to understand ASL without any instruction. In fact, ASL has a full capacity to express abstract concepts that cannot be directly pictured.

When new terms are needed, sign languages may borrow from each other and from spoken languages, just as spoken languages do (Battison, 1978). There is no reason to believe that the vocabulary of ASL is either limited or primitive.

ASL has evolved in directions that turn out to be predictable. Many signs that were originally pictorial have become less so, signs have shifted to positions in which they are more visible, two-handed signs made near the face have tended to become one-handed, and two-handed signs made at a distance from the face have become more symmetrical (Klima and Bellugi, 1979).

Words (spoken, written, or signed) are related to the concepts they express. Signed and spoken words may have very different meanings, or several signs may be used for one English word, and vice versa. The criticism sometimes encountered that sign languages are concept-based rather than word-based is incorrect; *all* languages are concept-based.

Fingerspelling is almost always used in combination with signing. *Name-signs* for people or places are like nicknames in spoken languages; they may incorporate a fingerspelled letter. (For example, Roger the physician may have a name-sign consisting of the letter "r" at the wrist in the same position as the sign for "doctor.") Short fingerspelled words may be shortened still further or modified to become a new sign. Another process is *initializing*. Several closely related English words may be rendered with the same sign using a different fingerspelled letter as part of the hand-shape ("*t*ry," "*e*ffort," and "*a*ttempt," for example).

Through the use of space, ASL has many ways of expressing meaning. As Klima and Bellugi (1979) have said:

> . . . if sound constitutes such a natural signal for language, then it is all the more striking how the human mind, when deprived of the faculty that makes sound accessible, seizes on, perfects, and systematizes an alternate form to enable the deeper linguistic faculties to give explicit expression to ideas. [p. 315]

Other signing codes include so-called *home signs*, developed within a family and unrelated to the signing of deaf adults (Goldin-Meadow and Feldman, 1975); *school signs*, used within a particular school; *childrenese*, a modified pidgin used by schoolchildren; and *local signs*, which vary in different parts of a country, like a dialect.

EFFICIENCY

Klima and Bellugi (1979) have reported some very helpful findings on ASL. The speed at which you can get your message across to another person is about the same in ASL and English. As soon as English sentences are coded into signs in a manually coded system, speed drops considerably. This is because the ways in which ASL uses space and motion are not employed to the same extent (or sometimes not at all). It may be that this relative slowness is one factor working against the adoption of a manually coded oral language as a native language for deaf people (Charrow, 1976).

EMOTIONAL EXPRESSIVENESS

Sign languages are well adapted to express emotions. This is one characteristic that gives considerable pleasure to many hearing learners. What a spoken language may do with volume, pitch, intonation, and other devices, sign languages do with space and movement.

Klima and Bellugi (1979) also give an excellent discussion (with pictures) of wit and poetry in ASL. Humor expressed in signs and mime is, of course, that which is appropriate to a visual-gestural language. Many sign language idioms are different from those in the spoken language of the same country. Sign language puns are not plays on the *sounds* of words, but on *visual* aspects of signs. For example, the sign for New York City, made with one hand on top of the palm of the other, can be made upside-down, visually indicating various negative meanings. Much humor based upon speech is lost in a sign language, and vice versa.

In the United States, the National Theater of the Deaf has developed drama, using ASL, to a highly artistic level. This professional group, consisting mostly of deaf actors and actresses, makes international tours and plays to audiences of deaf and hearing people. There are also deaf professional and amateur theater groups in several other countries, and in several local areas in North America.

HOW EASY IS IT TO LEARN A SIGN LANGUAGE?

For deaf children, learning a sign language is no more difficult than for a hearing child to learn any spoken language. When sign language is constantly used around deaf or hearing children, their own skills in the language develop at about the same rate as speech does with hearing children—or sometimes earlier because less fine coordination is needed for signs than for speech (Holmes and Holmes, 1980; Schlesinger, 1978a).

Hearing adults usually find it hard work to learn *any* new language, and sign languages are no exception, contrary to some popular opinion. The belief that learning a sign language is easy is a dangerous myth; if you do not realize this, you may become easily discouraged. Fingerspelling is another matter; the letters can be learned in a few minutes or an hour, but proficiency in *reading* rapid fingerspelling when it is interspersed with signing is much more difficult to acquire. A manual code or pidgin is easier for hearing people to learn than a native sign language. Because your child is very likely to become a user of your country's native sign language, we believe it is of fundamental importance to *appreciate* the language, even though you should not expect to become a fluent user without a great deal of motivation and hard work. Modern techniques of second-language teaching and learning are being applied to ASL; it is possible that easier ways for hearing persons to learn it will soon be available.

A pidgin form of sign language, such as PSE, has certain advantages in that it is more flexible than manual codes; therefore, more native sign language forms can be incorporated into it as one's experience increases.

The following are examples of common but very misleading ideas about the ease of learning sign languages:

> . . . to my surprise, I found that learning the sign language wasn't anything like as difficult and complicated as I had previously thought [p. 7] . . . . it is not as intimidating as it might appear at first. Because it is a visual language, there are no complicated grammatical rules to learn, no awkward tenses and no difficult declensions. [Jones and Willis, 1972, p. 10]

> Sign language is a kind of a shorthand using the hands and facial expressions. It is not a translation of English words, but simply conveys simple concepts without tenses or grammar or shades of meaning. [Mackey and Heilman, 1978, p. 150]

In a book on sign and gesture languages or systems, the famous British neurologist Macdonald Critchley (1975) shows similar errors, first when he discusses the sign system used by different North American Indian tribes, then when he supports the idea that all deaf people instinctively know how to sign:

> Indians can communicate without any difficulty with the deaf of any nationality [p. 71] . . . all deaf-mutes possess another and lesser known system which is a kind of manual shorthand, whereby a simple gesture stands not for a letter but for a word, a phrase, or even a sentence. [p. 57]

EFFECTS ON SPOKEN AND
WRITTEN LANGUAGE DEVELOPMENT

There is evidence that the early use of a sign language or sign code does not retard spoken language development if speech and auditory training are given sufficient attention as components of a Total Communication program (Schlesinger, 1978a and 1978b; Vernon and Koh, 1970, 1971).

DEAF PERSONS AS SIGN LANGUAGE INSTRUCTORS

Although we believe that hearing people generally learn a sign language better from a deaf teacher than in any other way, deafness does not automatically make someone a competent instructor. Neither should every deaf adult be expected to act as an expert on the structure or vocabulary of sign language. We don't expect hearing persons to do this for spoken languages.

WHAT IS TAUGHT IN A "SIGN LANGUAGE COURSE"?

Courses in sign language have become much more widely available. However, you should be aware of what you are getting, because the courses are not usually in *sign language*. Instead, you will probably be learning *sign vocabulary*, in which signs are put together in the word order of the spoken language (similar to PSE), perhaps with the addition of some features of a manually coded system. There is nothing wrong with this system as long as it is recognized as such. Taking such a course will not by itself enable you to fully understand a native sign language, but it will assist you in learning to communicate with those deaf people who can use this form of signing.

APES AND AMERICAN SIGN LANGUAGE

Several apes have been reported to learn and to use ASL after many years of training by American investigators. It is true that the apes do use signs, but they are not using ASL, and it is now doubted by some that they are really creating signed sentences (Terrace et al., 1979). There is a danger in these reports apart from their scientific interest—that the old idea of sign language being primitive will thereby be reinforced.

DEVELOPMENT OF TECHNICAL SIGNS

New signs, like new words in English, are needed for new kinds of technology, events, or situations. Insofar as possible, these signs should be chosen to be compatible with related signs and to suit the grammatical patterns of the particular sign language concerned.

CONCLUSION

Sign languages are receiving greatly increased attention, but much still remains to be learned. ASL is the only language that has been moderately well investigated; study of the others is only beginning.

SUMMARY

1. Feelings about sign language tend to be very emotional and strongly held, but they are often based upon misconceptions.

2. Parents should have a basic understanding of what sign languages are, how they compare with oral languages and sign codes, and what the effects of using one of these languages or systems for their deaf child may be.

3. Cued speech is not a sign language, but a manual system to aid in speechreading. It seems to have some benefit for this purpose, but it is doubtful that it can provide early enough two-way communication.

4. Fingerspelling is a way of writing in the air, not an independent language. It may be combined with speech in the Rochester Method, but it is slow and of doubtful value as a first language for deaf children. Fingerspelling is used to supplement sign language for proper names and to express concepts for which signs are not known.

5. Sign languages are true languages with their own structure. There is no universal sign language. Deaf people also use mime to enhance their expressiveness, but this should not be confused with rule-governed sign language.

6. Native sign languages are no easier for hearing people to learn than any foreign language.

7. Deaf children are unique in that most of them acquire sign language from their peers rather than from their parents, who are not usually signers. Young hearing children, however, have access to adult and to child models for language development.

8. We all automatically change our way of communicating in response to different situations (code-switching). This is also true of child and adult users of sign languages.

9. There are gradations (a continuum) from a pure

native sign language at one extreme to a form
close to the structure of the oral language at the
other. Between these two extremes there are
mixed forms called pidgins, which develop
naturally when two languages are in contact
with each other. This has happened with
American Sign Language and English, and the
combination is known as Pidgin Sign English or
PSE.

10. American Sign Language (ASL) is the most-
studied of all sign languages.

11. Manually coded systems have been invented in
several countries to parallel the structure of the
oral or spoken language. Most of these systems
(of which there are several in North America)
use the vocabulary of their native sign language.
They are used mostly by teachers and by hearing
parents, but not by many deaf adults. (Some
invented signs have been assimilated into ASL.)

12. In practice, there is a fair degree of mutual
intelligibility between parents who learn a
manually coded form of signing and those deaf
persons who can code-switch closer to the
spoken-language form.

13. Close study of ASL has shown that the old ideas
about its deficiencies are wrong. It is fully able
to express abstract concepts and fine shades of
meaning. Space and motion are used in place of
the word-endings and changes of basic words
(inflections) that are used in oral languages.

14. Coding English into signs and invented sign-
endings slows the rate of transmission of
information.

15. Sign languages express emotion, wit, poetry,
and humor in their own unique ways.

16. Most courses in "sign language" are courses in
sign vocabulary or a pidgin sign language.
Parents should not expect to become fluent in a
native sign language without considerable and
prolonged effort.

17. There is much doubt that apes can learn and use ASL as has been reported in the past. They can, however, learn sign vocabulary.
18. Technical signs for use in academic and other special settings have been developed, but these new signs should first be subjected to study so that the ones chosen suit the grammar and vocabulary of that sign language.
19. There is no sign code or sign language that is conclusively known to best suit all deaf children. The establishment of early and pleasurable two-way communication is essential; the form this communication takes is of secondary importance.

Chapter 12

TOTAL COMMUNICATION
Putting It All Together

INTRODUCTION

There are many misconceptions surrounding the term "Total Communication." The definition often quoted is:

> Total Communication implies that the congenitally deaf child must be introduced early in life to a reliable receptive-expressive system of symbols which he is free to learn to manipulate for himself and from which he can abstract meaning in the course of unrestricted interaction with other persons. Total Communication includes the full spectrum of language modes: child-devised gestures, the language of signs, speech, speechreading, fingerspelling, reading and writing. Total Communication incorporates the development of any remnant of residual hearing for the enhancement of speech and speechreading skills through long-term consistent use of individual hearing aids and/or high fidelity group amplification systems. [Denton, 1976, p. 4]

The term "Total Communication" was probably first used in this way by a deaf teacher, Dr. Roy Holcomb. The concept was first fully implemented by him in Santa Ana (California) and by Dr. David Denton at the Maryland School for the Deaf. (Denton led in the movement to promote Total Communication internationally.)

It is important to distinguish Total Communication, as a flexible approach, from a specific set of techniques applicable to every deaf child. Until fairly recently, education for deaf children was of two major kinds: *pure oral* (oral-only) and the *combined method* (auditory/oral with signs and fingerspelling added). The great majority of schools (both day programs and residential) advocated the oral-only approach, officially banning the use of signs. Outside the classroom, however, the oral children signed to each other, despite disapproval.

Although Total Communication includes the use of residual hearing, speech, fingerspelling, and signing, it should not, in our view, he referred to as a new version of the old term "combined method," as some oralist critics maintain (Meadow, 1980). It embraces this combination as appropriate to many educational situations, but Total Communication can also involve improving hearing and speech (with or without signing), the development of miming skills to enhance the child's expressiveness, and the introduction of signing in infancy, long before school entrance. (In Australia our description would still be called the combined method.)

The major benefits of Total Communication are that it encourages the acceptance of the deaf child as a deaf person whose early language can grow rapidly in response to developing needs, and that it stresses an individualized approach according to the skills of each deaf child (Meadow, 1980; Mindel and Vernon, 1971; Moores, 1978b).

THE ORAL-MANUAL CONTROVERSY

Introduction

We do not wish to go into great detail about the oral-manual controversy, because there are many references and reviews elsewhere (Conrad, 1979; Lane, 1980; Meadow, 1980; Mindel and Vernon, 1971; Moores, 1978b; Royal National Institute for the Deaf, 1976). Neither can we ignore it, although Luterman (1979) suggests this would be best. It is important for parents and professional workers to have a basic understanding of the issues and assumptions involved in the dispute.

The Oralist Argument

As recently as 1972, Silverman, a well-known advocate of oral-only education, stated:

> It is *generally agreed* that sign language is *bound to the concrete* and is *limited* with respect to abstraction, humor, and subtleties, such as figures of speech which enrich expression. [p. 405, emphasis added]

Such uninformed statements are all too common from "experts," who neither know sign language nor the results of modern sign language research. This quotation could not be supported by anyone who "speaks" a sign language and who knows its richness and variety. It is time that claims like this disappeared from standard texts in deaf education, speech pathology, and audiology. In his discussion of the oral-manual controversy, Silverman concluded:

> Oralists feel that, in the main, orally trained children have done well and are likely to do better as more teachers are adequately trained in the methods of oral instruction. [p. 406]

Silverman has apparently modified these views, because one of his new books (Davis and Silverman, 1978) is much better balanced. Ling, an advocate of the auditory approach, stated: "There is no question that sign language is a viable language in its own right" (1978, p. 298). However, he rejects it as insufficient because of its lack of a parallel with speech and written language.

Total Communication advocates have allowed themselves to be forced into a strange position: they have accepted the challenge posed by the oralists to prove that the addition of fingerspelling and signs to auditory/oral techniques does not limit the deaf child's development of auditory/oral communication skills, reading, or writing. We say this is "strange" because the oralists (who have almost completely controlled deaf education for 100 years) have never supplied scientific follow-up support for their own restrictive approach (Conrad, 1979, 1980). However, as a result of accepting this challenge, there are now a respectable number of studies that are in general agreement. (These studies have been reviewed by Conrad, 1979.) The studies show that many of the assumptions of the oralists are without any solid foundation. (In the remainder of this chapter, when we refer to English, readers should understand that *any* spoken language could be substituted for English.)

Oralist Assumptions

1. *Total Communication is Taking the Easy Way Out.* If signing is introduced early, oralists claim, deaf children will not be motivated to work hard to acquire auditory/oral skills because signs are easier to learn (Ling, 1978).
2. *Signing and Sign Languages are Inadequate Communication Systems.* Oralists have considered sign languages to be limited, concrete, and primitive; many of them still do.
3. *Learning to Sign Enforces Segregation.* As a result of learning to sign, deaf children will drift into "the deaf world," losing the opportunity to participate fully in society. (This is argued even by those oralists, like Ling, who accept the fact that sign languages are languages.)

These three assumptions, which have caused many parents to feel threatened, have little basis in fact. Furthermore, the results of oral-only education, especially for prelingually deaf children, have been very poor, in spite of dominance by the oralists during a time of relatively lavish funding (Conrad, 1980; Furth, 1966; Meadow, 1980). As we have seen in previous chapters, the deaf children of deaf parents, most of whom have been signing since infancy, do at least as well as deaf children in oral-only programs in reading and auditory/oral skills (Conrad, 1979). The adequacy of sign languages was discussed in Chapter 11. In Chapter 2, we argued that life as a deaf person provides multiple opportunities to cross the boundaries of deaf and hearing groups. (Most deaf children will learn to sign even if they have been in oral-only programs.)

Concern for the future of deaf children, based upon the early need for communication, does not allow a calm, dispassionate discussion of these matters. One of the unspoken oralist assumptions is that the great delay in establishment of early communication is not a really serious matter; it is believed that the child will catch up. We believe this assumption to be wrong. The controversy has been likened to a religious war. Although there may be some similarities, this comparison is inaccurate. We are discussing not only a type of faith or dogma, but also facts and theories based upon the best evidence available (Benderly, 1980).

There are several unfortunate consequences of the oral-manual controversy: it puzzles, worries, and frustrates parents; it deprives many deaf children of the communicative richness in early childhood that is their right; and it sometimes has set deaf adults and hearing parents against each other, when they should be allies.

The Total Communication Position

Deaf children of deaf parents learn sign language naturally and quickly. Which is more "natural"–deaf children learning a system they can acquire easily and quickly (signing), even though their parents must learn to use a new mode, or struggling for years to use the mode of language their parents use, without any other options? Whatever the definition of "natural," we accept the oralists' complaint that sign language is easy for the deaf child to learn, and we rejoice in it. The "easy way out" is fine—it is not something to fear, and it is beneficial for the deaf child.

Because sign language use with young deaf children need not lead to a loss of other communication skills (provided these are given an opportunity to develop), because deaf children need a reliable early communication system, and because deaf people who sign are not segregated in a lonely "ghetto," the restrictive oral-only argument is without any firm foundation. However, potentially useful auditory-oral skills may be neglected by some Total Communication programs and by some parents whose enthusiasm for signing is not well balanced or individualized.

Other Similar Controversies

Deafness is not the only field in which there has been controversy over goals (either becoming like the majority *or* remaining segregated). A similar battle was fought over whether blind people should be allowed to use a separate (Braille) system of reading and writing; this conflict was known as "the war of the dots." Similarly, education of underprivileged black children in the United States was hampered for years by a false assumption that the language they were using was a defective version of Standard English that required remediation. It is now known that their dialect (Black English Vernacular) is a fully adequate variant of English that the teacher needs to understand before Standard English can be effectively taught. These and other examples have been briefly discussed by Freeman (1976).

In these and other similar instances, the majority view of the minority's way of functioning is distorted and unhelpful. The language of deaf people is also often treated in this way.

We have been highly critical of the oralists, but this does not mean that we do not appreciate some of the advances they have made, nor that we see them as less dedicated to the welfare of deaf children than are Total Communication advocates.

WHAT IS THE PRESENT
STATUS OF TOTAL COMMUNICATION?

Until recently it was typical for the use of signing to be permitted only after years of "oral failure" or only when the child left school. Deaf children grew up (and most still do) without the skill to communicate with their own families or to understand the intentions of their parents.

Led by the United States and by the Scandinavian countries, there has now been a massive shift from oral-only to Total Communication programs in both day and residential schools for deaf children (Garretson, 1976; Jordan, Gustason, and Rosen, 1979). In the United States, manually coded English has an important place in instruction at the preschool and primary levels. PSE is still widely used at the secondary level. ASL, however, has no official place in instruction (Kannapell, 1978).

In the United Kingdom, the influence of the oral teachings of Manchester University has been overwhelming until very recently. Starting in Scotland (Montgomery, 1976) and northern England at Newcastle-Upon-Tyne, Total Communication has arrived. It is now officially accepted in some Scottish and English day and residential schools, and is supported by the British Deaf Association and the National Union of the Deaf. The teachers' organization is still staunchly oral, however. The Royal National Institute for the Deaf, which formerly took no official position on the methods controversy, now in effect supports Total Communication, although the phrase is not mentioned by name (RNID, 1978). Readers in the United States may not fully appreciate how revolutionary the RNID change has been. The text of the unanimous policy statement is re-printed in the Appendix to this chapter.

Canada and Australia have various types of programs, depending upon the school and region of the country. Other parts of the (British) Commonwealth, all of which were strongly influenced by oralism, are changing at various rates. Malaysia, for example, has officially shifted to a Total Communication approach for young deaf children. A manually coded Malay system, adapted from ASL, is being devised (there is apparently no native sign language). Malay has few inflections, so that a manually coded form may be quite successful (Tan Chin Guan, personal communication, 1980).

France, famous as a major historic source of ASL, is strictly oral, but interest in Total Communication is increasing.

It seems that all, or nearly all, recent changes have been in the direction of Total Communication, although we have been informed that Italy is closing all of its schools for deaf children in favor of mainstreaming (Conrad, personal communication, 1980).

MUST SIGNS AND SPEECH
ALWAYS BE USED TOGETHER?

Many persons who advocate a Total Communication philosophy believe that signs and speech must always be used together:

> It (signing) is, of course, always used simultaneously with speech, thus signing reinforces speechreading and speechreading reinforces signing and better communication is the result. [Denton, 1976, p. 4]
> . . . residual hearing, speech, speechreading, signs, fingerspelling, and gestures are used simultaneously in communication. [IAPD, 1976, p. 9]

Although in many situations oral and manual modes are appropriately used together, we do not believe that this must always be insisted upon. Perhaps instead the requirement of simultaneity should be re-examined.

We have argued that a native sign language has an important place in a deaf child's linguistic and social development, but it cannot be easily used to parallel the spoken language, because its structure is different. If we believe that ASL (for example) is an adequate language, then why not use it fully and joyfully (when the persons concerned can) and stop feeling guilty about not speaking simultaneously? To define a sign language only as a "supplement" to oral language is to relegate it to a second-class position; this seems antagonistic to the principles of Total Communication.

Manual codes and pidgins, however, can be used simultaneously when speaking *to* children who are deaf. We may also encourage deaf children to speak when they sign; but if their speech is very poor, the insistence upon simultaneous expression by the children could inhibit their self-expression. It seems that the rules need to be sensibly applied to a child's individual situation.

A rigid approach is unnecessary and probably damaging. There is a likelihood that deaf children will come to feel that signing is second best if they are taught that speaking and listening are all-important and that these skills should *never* be omitted. At the same time they can see that signing is not done by many hearing people and not even by some deaf people and therefore it can apparently be omitted. Deaf children should be developing their own judgment of what form of communication is appropriate so that they can code- or mode-switch depending upon the person, topic, and situation. It is this flexibility of application that makes Total Communication desirable.

We suspect that one possible reason for the rigid insist- ence upon constant simultaneous usage of signs with speech in schools is political and ideological—it "looks good" to some parents, visitors, and government officials. Combined oral-manual use also proves that the program isn't a "man- ual" program, as some oralists would accuse it of being. The time has come to be frank. Big risks have been taken with the lives of deaf children and their families for many years. We should be willing to accept the risk that some unknow- ledgeable critics will call us "manualists." If the child's needs, not the system, really determine the form of communication, then we should not need to be defensive.

ARE THERE LIMITATIONS TO SIGNING?

Like any other form of communication, signing has advan- tages and disadvantages. Its full use requires adequate vision and both hands, so it is less useful in the dark or when both hands are fully occupied. Also, unlike hearing, you must pay visual attention to the signer. It should be pointed out, however, that it is not necessary to put down the things you are carrying in order to sign. Even two-handed signs can be made with one hand; the other hand's movement can be understood from context.

In the midst of controversy another "limitation" may be almost forgotten: *the use of signs or sign language does not solve all of life's problems for deaf children!* They can have all of the

difficulties any child can have. Using signs or sign language
is a very effective way of equalizing risks and problems, not
of preventing all of them.

UNSETTLED ISSUES

Total Communication advocates do not agree on everything,
and there is no reason why they should, any more than
professionals do in other areas of educational or medical
practice. In this section, a few issues of disagreement are
discussed in relation to prelingually deaf children. Children
who become deaf postlingually usually need all or many of
the components of Total Communication, but the maintenance of already established spoken communication is a high
priority.

What System of Manual
Communication Should be Introduced at the Start?

Hearing parents cannot usually learn a native sign language
quickly enough to use it with their very young deaf child, so
a form approximating English is ordinarily chosen, but
which type? Should it be a manual English code or PSE?
Different answers can be offered. We ourselves use PSE and
do not worry about absolute uniformity, especially because
deaf children are usually very adept at adjusting their
language, or *code-switching* (Schlesinger, 1978a and 1978b).
We prefer PSE to a manual code because it is more flexible
(Reilly and McIntire, 1980). We would have no objections to
parents using a manual code so long as they acknowledge
the existence of, and appreciate, ASL. (The Paget-Gorman
Sign System favored by some in the United Kingdom would
be excluded by us as a possibility because it blocks social
access to the deaf community.)

The use of a pidgin sign language with the minimum
of new signs to bring it close to English, will not, so far as we
know, prevent deaf children from learning and using English

grammar and structure in their spoken or written language. Further follow-up research would be helpful on this question.

How Can the Type of Sign System Used at Home be Linked With That Used in the School?

Parents sometimes start asking how to link the home sign system with that used in the school as soon as they become aware of the school's policy on sign language and sign codes. They worry that their child will be confused. Perhaps they do not give deaf children enough credit for their ability to code-switch. We do not believe it is essential to use a manual code in an early intervention or preschool program just because a manual code will be used later in elementary school.

Bilingualism

The way to make deaf children proud of themselves is intimately linked with the dignity given to their language and to their way of communicating. As Paul (1973) has stated: "The deaf person who is truly bilingual, and who knows both Ameslan and English is rarely encouraged to be equally proud of both" (p. 41). There have not yet been enough opportunities or enough time to see the results of trying to build pride. Those oralists who claim that sign language was always used in residential schools, and that therefore Total Communication is nothing new, have totally missed the point. In those schools signing was forbidden, punished, sometimes tolerated, but almost never welcomed and encouraged to flourish from the child's earliest years in a bilingual environment. Even today the question of how to use a native sign language creatively in a school is largely untried and unanswered.

Without claiming to have all the answers, we advocate the exposure of young deaf children to native sign language users. It is even better if there is a recognized place for native sign language within the school program. This is not to suggest that all classes should be taught in ASL. Once the decision is made to use it, however, many ideas will be generated by students, teachers, and deaf adults. It is this kind of bilingualism that is especially needed.

One way of providing a bilingual environment has been described by Erting (1978) and has been used in a number of preschools (including ours): a native signer is hired as teacher or aide.

In What Way, and at What Time, Should Auditory/Oral Training be Introduced?

Although Total Communication includes the techniques of auditory/oral training, we want to avoid mutilating the deaf child's self-esteem by overfocussing on what he or she cannot do or can only do poorly. Therefore, it is necessary to accept deafness as a difference rather than as a deficit to be corrected. From this principle, we can derive the concept that attention to hearing aid use, to auditory training, and to training in speech and speechreading should be provided in a way that does not overemphasize the child's deficiencies. Simply talking to the child while signing is not adequate. Although we wish to develop language as naturally as possible, it may be advisable to have special sessions in the use of amplification and in speech, rather than constantly correcting the child's speech throughout the day. However, too much enthusiasm for sign language can obscure the real benefits that some children derive from amplification. (We can never afford to forget that deaf children with similar audiograms may make very different use of amplification.) We hope for further developments in this area as experience is broadened.

HOW CAN YOU JUDGE THE ADEQUACY OF A TOTAL COMMUNICATION PROGRAM?

A successful Total Communication program calls for teachers and other staff who enjoy communicating with deaf children and adults in signs or in sign language, and who know and respect the deaf community. Parents who still have problems accepting their child's deafness will need sympathetic counseling as well as assistance in learning how to communicate with their child.

Auditory/oral components should not be taken for granted, but their place needs to be carefully thought out. Negative consequences of repeated failure should be considered. Hearing aids should be kept in good working order, and auditory training equipment must be properly maintained.

Deaf adults should be involved in the teaching process (Ladd, 1978; Merrill, 1979). They can provide role models and native sign language experience.

The following list of questions has been modified from suggestions for successful programs received from our resource persons. It is meant to guide your own assessments, not to be all-inclusive or to set absolute standards.

1. Is there easy communication and social interaction among the children and staff? Are children under stress because they find it difficult to communicate?
2. Considering communication, are children frequently corrected, or are they encouraged to express themselves freely?
3. Are the staff's attitudes toward deafness and toward deaf children positive?
4. Are deaf adults involved in the program so that the children can interact with them?
5. Are there enough children in the program to provide a wide variety of social opportunities?
6. Is there excessive emphasis placed upon speech and hearing, or is there a reasonable balance with non-speech communication?
7. Is there a place for the native sign language, or is only a manual code allowed? Is the environment flexible enough for a variety of communication modalities to flourish?
8. Are the children permitted to do things that are age-appropriate, or are they overprotected and perhaps considered incompetent?
9. Are there free play and activities available that are *fun* and

Table 3. Options for Communication

Group	Native Sign Language	Pidgin or Sign Code	Auditory/Oral Training	Deaf Community
Prelingual onset of profound deafness; with deaf parents	Usually the first language	Will be used as route for second language learning	Should be tried as supplement	Usually automatic
Prelingual onset of profound deafness; with hearing parents	Probably learned later as second language	Usual route for acquiring first language	Should be tried; rarely adequate for first language	Essential
Substantial hearing for speech	Variable; can't hurt and may be helpful	May be a second mode	May be adequate for first language	Variable
Late or postlingual onset with hearing parents	May be learned as second language later	Important as second mode for first language	Essential to preserve skills in first language	Variable
Multiply handicapped deaf; hearing parents	Probably will not be learned	May be useful; or simplified system may be needed	Should be tried, but unlikely to be enough	Variable
Diagnosis late or program late	May be learned as second language	Likely will be route for first language	Should be tried; but unlikely to be enough	Essential

that are appropriate to the child's developmental level, or are children forced into constant work and drill?

10. Do academic activities excite, intellectually challenge, and actively involve the children, or do they encourage boredom and passivity?
11. Is attention given to improving the parents' communication skills?
12. Is sympathetic counseling available for those parents who need it?
13. Is the entire family involved in the program, or is no effort made to actively involve both parents, siblings, and relatives?
14. Are the premises adequately treated for protection from excessive noise? Is auditory training equipment well maintained?
15. Are deaf people represented on the staff, administration, and Board of Directors?

CONCLUSIONS

As Naiman and Schein (1978) have said:

> Do not let communication become a battleground. Avoid emotional appeals to choose the one best way. Communication is too important for such decisions. Your child needs to know what you are thinking and feeling, and you need to understand your child. That is the prime issue before which all others must give way. [1978, p. 23]

We would add that parents must accept their child's deafness, the overriding need for communication and language (which are more important than speech), and the need to gain satisfaction from a mutual and warm relationship. A good Total Communication program should facilitate all of the above needs, and should offer each child and family the options uniquely suited to their situation. (A summary of our view of these options is in Table 3.)

SUMMARY

1. There are many misconceptions about Total Communication. It involves flexible use, from the earliest possible time, of all important means of communication, not a specific set of techniques for all deaf children.

2. Because of the long-standing oral-manual controversy, Total Communication advocates have been challenged to justify their approach. Fears of the bad effects of signing have been shown to be unfounded—signing deaf children need not give up their attempts at speech if they have the capacity to acquire it. Sign languages are not defective languages. Their use does not enforce segregation.

3. For most prelingually deaf children, the results of oral-only education have been quite poor.

4. In other fields the majority has also tried to force a minority to do things their way, with unfortunate results.

5. Total Communication is spreading worldwide. It is now the predominant approach for deaf children in the United States. Major changes are occurring in Canada, England, Scotland, and in other countries.

6. Although signs and speech should often be used together (simultaneous communication), a flexible Total Communication program does not exclude the use of one form of communicating without the other if the circumstances warrant this.

7. Although non-speech communication is ordinarily very easy for deaf children to acquire, it will not in itself solve or prevent all problems.

8. There are as yet unsettled issues in Total Communication: 1) what system of non-speech communication to adopt for hearing parents, 2) how non-oral communication should be linked with the system used by the child's

school, and 3) how best to include auditory/oral components in Total Communication programs.

9. Amplification, auditory training, and speech can be used differently with each deaf child. The potential benefits of these components of Total Communication should not be ignored as a result of the enthusiasm for signs.

10. A list of questions is provided in this chapter to guide observations of Total Communication programs and to assess their quality. Emphasis is placed on the active involvement of the whole family in learning to communicate freely and fully with the child; on the participation of deaf adults; on the acceptance of deafness as a difference, rather than a deficit; and on the attitudes of the teaching staff toward deafness, deaf people, the language of signs, and freedom of communication.

APPENDIX TO CHAPTER 12

Methods of education of deaf children have been the subject of detailed and searching discussion within the Institute and, at its meeting on 16th March, 1978, the Council unanimously adopted the following statement as its expression of policy:

Most profoundly deaf children, even with modern methods of amplification of speech and lipreading, do not make satisfactory educational and social progress. This is acknowledged by many teachers and others involved with the education and care of deaf children and the RNID held a Seminar followed later by a Conference on the methods of communication currently used in the education of deaf children.

The consensus of opinion expressed at both the Seminar and Conference was:

(a) in favour of a liberal approach to methods of communication in the education and care of deaf children;

(b) that parents of deaf children should have the opportunity to

acquire skills in manual communication, as well as in other methods:

       and

(c)   instruction in manual communication should be included in all training programmes for teachers of deaf children.

The Institute has found no evidence that the addition of manual methods is likely to inhibit the development of oral skills. It advises parents of deaf children not to be deterred by statements which cast doubt on the efficacy of these methods: failure to develop effective parent/child communication in the vital early years will seriously retard the general progress of deaf children.

The RNID accepts the consensus of opinion expressed at the Seminar and Conference and urges those responsible for the training of teachers of deaf children to include in their training programmes adequate instruction in manual communication in addition to auditory training, lip reading and the teaching of speech.

Chapter 13

RAISING A DEAF CHILD

It is extremely sad when a mother with a genuine loving concern for her child is made to feel she is no use to him. In fact in those cases where mothers did give up with their children it was often because they were made to feel inadequate—and made to feel it was a job for experts. [Gregory, 1976, p. 132]

Somehow when my child was diagnosed as deaf, I stopped seeing him as a child and looked at him as DEAF . . . I believe we can prevent mismanagement in childhood if we all learn to respect the deaf child as a person, to listen to him, to learn from him, and to share with him. This means we must learn to communicate with him on his terms, and to understand his behavior as communication. [Wilson, 1976, p. 29]

INTRODUCTION

Giving advice on child-rearing is easy, and there is no shortage of experts. Advice is usually based, however, upon several wrong assumptions: that there actually is a body of factual knowledge about the best child-rearing techniques, that these techniques can be taught, and that teaching the techniques to parents will be beneficial to their children. Bruch (1954) has warned about the dangerous "illusion of omnipotence" held by many parent-educators:

Whatever the psychological advice, one can be sure that it will be put into practice in as many different ways as there are parents [p. 726]. . . . the enumeration of all the possible acts and attitudes that might injure a child creates an atmosphere of uncertainty and apprehension [p. 727] . . . an outside authority, the family expert, stands watch and censures parents for possible errors and faults. It has made child care something akin to being sick and the necessary authority of parents has been undermined. They are no longer masters in their own homes, who raise their children in a way that seems right and proper to them. If the children have problems and encounter difficulty in living, the parents take the blame for having used the wrong method or having misunderstood the instruction [pp. 727–728]. . . . the child has been relegated to the position of being merely an indicator of the correctness of the theoretical conviction of some expert, or of the parent's perfection in putting it into practice. [p. 728]

When you have a deaf child, your sense of parental competence can be impaired by conflicting or insensitive advice. Although this chapter contains some discussion of child-rearing, it is not intended to set any generally applicable standards. It seems appropriate that hearing parents should get the same enjoyment from their deaf child as deaf parents do: through acceptance, easy communication, and a balance that satisfies everyone's needs. A particularly apt phrase used by Naiman and Schein (1978, p. 2) suggests that the proper focus on a deaf child in the family is as "a part, but not the center."

The subjects considered in this chapter include the impact of deafness on the family, personality development, behavior problems, opportunities for learning, social relationships, the community, and how to deal with the need for special help.

IMPACT OF DEAFNESS ON THE FAMILY

Effects on the Parents

A child with special needs poses challenges to any family's integrity. It is usually the mother, however, who is most heavily burdened. The mother is usually the parent who visits the experts, who works hard with the child, and who undergoes the most changes in feeling and understanding. Luterman (1979) has stated that most "parent education" is really "mother education." If the father works during the day, it is more difficult for him to participate in activities that take place during working hours. He is less likely to visit professionals or clinics with his child. Gradually the mother becomes relatively better informed. An imbalance in family roles can result.

Some of the recommendations we professionals make can place parents in uncomfortable or unwelcome positions. For example, by "instructing" them we may remind them of unpleasant school experiences. We are concerned that even within this chapter, by pointing out potential problem areas, we may increase some parents' worries. Finding out how to do everything to the recommended extent and yet to balance everyone's needs, including your own, is a great challenge! There are no simple formulas: "Raising children was, is, and always will be a mission of love. . . . Basically, what is indispensable to our children is learning to live in harmony with themselves and others. This cannot be accomplished by a technical process" (Anonymous, 1979, p. 1). One of our resource persons commented:

> . . . finding a balance is itself an ongoing process . . . involving daily difficult choices, not one brilliant decision arrived at one day. . . . The important thing is not to add to the body of literature that makes us feel guilty about one thing or another. . . . I personally feel tired of being criticized for whatever role I take and being told at the same time not to feel inadequate.

If the parents had marriage problems before their child arrived, the deaf child's presence may aggravate these problems. Overall, however, separation and divorce are not more common among parents of deaf children. These findings were reported in 1975 (Freeman et al.), and studies of families whose children have other disabilities have confirmed this report (Fundudis, Kolvin, and Garside, 1979; Jan et al., 1977). Although there is no study directly comparable to the Vancouver study of the families of deaf children, the Vancouver finding is indirectly supported by Schlesinger and Meadow (1972) and by Gregory (1976). In both of these other studies, parents were asked how the presence of the deaf child had affected their marriages. The replies were about equally divided between good and bad effects. (It should be noted that separation and divorce are only crude measures of the impact of a deaf child on a marriage.)

In raising a deaf child, financial burdens may also be increased. In some countries medical care, hearing aids, and hearing aid batteries can require a considerable sum of money. The family may have to move to be closer to a special school or other services, and may have to pay for certain special programs.

Angry feelings toward your child are a natural result of frustration. Many parents wish, at times, that their child had never been born. Deaf children are more frustrating than hearing children because hopes and goals seem less clear and feelings of guilt are more likely.

> Mr. and Mrs. A. had serious problems with their marriage for several years. Both were rather young and still dependent upon their own parents' approval. Mrs. A became increasingly bitter as she took Jack to visit doctors and audiologists and then became actively involved in a parent organization, while her husband felt he was adequately performing his role as a good provider—period. Her frustrations resulted in frequent spankings of Jack, which reminded Mr. A of his own unhappy childhood experiences. He was convinced that his wife was having a "nervous breakdown" because of her devotion to the cause of deafness. Arguing increased. The grandparents, realizing that things were amiss, tried to help. Their suggestions only aggravated the conflict. Soon Mrs. A began to feel that she was inadequate as a wife and daughter as well as as a mother because her husband seemed uninterested in her latest efforts and started coming home later at night. Only after a period of assessment could they identify some of the forces that had started to poison their relationship.

Why does it seem to be more difficult to discipline a deaf child? Can you be sure that the child understands you? Perhaps not. Can you tolerate seeing his or her feelings hurt? This may be painful. Do you (or your relatives) feel sorry for him or her? Do friends or relatives criticize you for the way you set limits, perhaps suggesting that you are hard-hearted? These are only a few of the possible complications. Uncertainty about discipline tends to highlight differences in style between mothers and fathers. These differences need to be resolved sufficiently so that one parent does not undermine the authority of the other. Deaf children are just as opportunistic as others—they will take advantage of their parents if they can. Advice that seems reasonable is to set the same limits and expectations for deaf as for hearing children, *if* you are reasonably sure that they are equally able to understand.

Other parental concerns, drawn from requests for help received by the IAPD, have been summarized by Fairchild (1979).

Effects on Siblings

Brothers and sisters (siblings) may also be affected by your child's deafness. If too much attention is paid to the deaf child, normal rivalry and jealousy may be intensified. There are several ways in which problems may arise. Hostility may be shown directly; this is common in young children. Frequent battles may occur. A more indirect expression of the need for attention is for the hearing child to wish to be deaf, too:

> When our partially integrated preschool/day care center (in Vancouver) was first opened, the enrollment consisted of several deaf children and one little hearing girl. She surprised her parents by requesting a hearing aid for Christmas!

It may be helpful to periodically assess whether your hearing children are receiving enough attention and encouragement. Resentment can occur and is best handled by seeking its source. If your hearing children are encouraged to reveal their feelings freely, it will be easier to discover whether a problem exists. (Much the same recommendation could be given for treating deaf children, too.)

A still more indirect manifestation of attention seeking is excessive devotion to the parents' cause (deafness), so that the hearing sibling becomes a kind of substitute parent. The hearing child may feel that the only way to gain acceptance is to enter the field of deafness later as a professional. How is it possible to tell whether a hearing child's interest in deafness is excessive? One indication is the suppression of *all* normal hostility and rivalry. Another sign is when the hearing child's interests are deliberately and repeatedly sacrificed. There is nothing wrong with sacrifice, but no ordinary deaf child benefits from being treated as if he were helpless or unable to tolerate any frustration. At the start, young brothers or sisters may not realize what is expected of them and may overdo for their deaf sibling, just as relatives may. It is really a question of whether the deaf child is truly made a member of the family. If a normal family relationship exists, then no one will be expected to be perfect or to always give up things in favor of anyone else.

A study of 77 hearing siblings of deaf children by Schwirian (1976) showed no ill effects from the presence of a deaf child. They were comparable to other hearing children chosen as a comparative group.

When hearing siblings enter adolescence, they may respond to the increased need to conform to their peer group by not wanting to associate with a deaf brother or sister. This is hard for some parents to understand, but the situation is usually temporary. It is generally thought best to discuss this problem openly, but not to attempt to enforce different behavior and values by imposing guilt feelings on the hearing child.

Effects on Relatives

Relatives may be an important source of support for parents, and they may also supply emotional warmth and wisdom to deaf children. However, relatives may also be a serious problem. Grandparents are often in a dilemma: although they feel sympathy for their own children (the deaf child's parents) and for their grandchild, they have little opportunity to participate in the experiences that gradually lead to parental acceptance of deafness. They usually have no (or outmoded) knowledge of deafness, and their responsibility for their deaf grandchild may be limited to baby-sitting. It is not surprising that many grandparents remain at the level of denying deafness or searching for miraculous cures. It is then difficult for the child's parents (who are still children to their own parents) simultaneously to maintain good relationships with their child, with each other, with the experts, and with the grandparents. (Similar situations may obtain for other relatives.)

We have found, as has Luterman (1979), that it is wise for professionals to inquire about the importance of relatives to each family. What are relatives' attitudes toward deafness and toward the management methods advised? Have their relationships with the parents changed for better or for worse? It often seems worthwhile to involve important relatives in some contacts with professionals, providing that this is desired by all concerned. It is unfortunate that efforts of this kind are so rarely made.

Need for Healthy Separation

Parents need their own time (individually, jointly, and with their other children) away from their deaf child and from deafness. Total absorption in deafness is not healthy, particularly when the level of involvement is very different for father and mother. Normally, children learn to tolerate separations gradually, through games (such as peek-a-boo and hide-and-seek) and through brief times away from their parents. If they have no such learning opportunities, children may have difficulty later in attending school or in allowing their parents to have a private life without giving major protest. It is healthy for children and parents to learn that they can survive without each other!

Greenberg and Marvin (1979) studied the separation behavior of 28 deaf children (average age 4½) who had hearing parents. Half of the children were in oral-only programs, and half were in Total Communication. Few real separation problems were seen. It may be of interest that the mothers who had children in oral-only programs used a meaningful sign to indicate to their children to wait and that mother would return. This was more effective than their extended spoken explanations.

Should You Have More Children?

An issue that sometimes arises with parents of deaf children is whether to have more children, a complex and individual matter. In the Vancouver study (Freeman et al., 1975), the families of 120 deaf children and of 120 matched hearing children were compared. Although many of the parents of deaf children reported that they had delayed having another child or avoided it altogether (because of the deaf child), as a group they had just as many additional children as did the parents of hearing children. Probably the most important consideration is not to make a decision that is hasty. Some outside advice, such as genetic counseling may be useful (see Chapter 5).

From Crisis to Crisis

Weathering one crisis in your child's development is no guarantee that there will be none later. Painful feelings that you thought were "settled" may return later (at times like school entry or adolescence), but they are usually temporary.

The essential thing to remember is that your deaf child can be a source of much pleasure and joy despite occasional crises.

The Parent's Role as Teacher

Different opinions have been expressed on the question whether it is good for a parent to take on a teaching role with his or her child, which often occurs with deaf children. A global judgment is impossible here, because there are so many differences in what, how, and how much is being taught. Luterman (1979) points out that all parents are teachers for their children. This is true, but perhaps it is worthwhile to ask oneself: Am I altering my natural relationship with my child? Am I overemphasizing deficiencies? Is the focus too much on "correct" forms of language rather than on communication? Am I neglecting my other children, my spouse, myself? In the final analysis, the guideline of Naiman and Schein (1978) may be simplest: "What is not good for the rest of the family is not good for the deaf child" (p. 3).

Deaf Parents

Deaf parents seem to be less affected emotionally by a diagnosis of deafness in their child than hearing parents are. Deaf parents may even have more problems raising a hearing child. In some cases, they overuse the child as an interpreter, but this is probably less of a difficulty now that professional interpreters are more widely available, and deaf parents are more aware of the negative effects on their hearing child.

PERSONALITY AND BEHAVIOR

Introduction

Personality grows in deaf children as it does in all children. Why, then, are there so many negative descriptions of the "typical deaf personality"? Deaf people are said to be emotionally immature, impulsive, egocentric, and lacking in feeling for others (Altshuler et al., 1976). In fact, it does appear that deaf children and adults are more likely to act impulsively than hearing people. (To act "impulsively" means to act on one's immediate feelings, without reflection and consideration.)

Explanations for Impulsivity

Three general kinds of explanations have been offered for impulsivity in deaf persons:

Damage to the brain. Some workers feel that many deaf children suffer brain damage through the same factors that caused their deafness. However, only a small proportion of deaf children show definite evidence of brain damage. Even if it is present, brain damage is not associated with any specific type of psychiatric disorder, although it increases the risk of all kinds of behavior problems.

Distortion of personality development because of lack of auditory input. Harris (1978) has shown that deaf children with deaf parents are significantly less likely to be overly impulsive than those with hearing parents. Therefore, impulsivity is not a universal or necessary result of deafness.

Deprivation of communication and incidental learning opportunities. We agree with Harris (1978) that deprivation of communication and of incidental learning opportunities seems to be the most likely explanation for impulsivity in deaf children.

It was originally thought that the differences in development that favor deaf children of deaf parents were because of a lesser likelihood of brain damage (and a greater likelihood that deafness was inherited) in this group. The research of Harris (1978) and of Conrad (1979) has disproven this. Early communication through sign language is probably one important factor favoring deaf children of deaf parents, but not necessarily the only one, because, on the average, deaf parents' attitudes toward their child's deafness is much more positive than is that of hearing parents.

New techniques are being developed to help impulsive children become more "reflective," but it seems wiser to build this into normal early development.

Temperament

It is obvious in the newborn nursery that children have different characteristics at birth: some are regular in feeding and sleeping, others are unpredictable; some are irritable and intense in their reactions, other babies tend to be placid. These patterns, known as temperament, are not unchangeable, but they do tend to persist. Although it used to be thought (and taught) that children's behavior is completely the result of how parents raise the child, this is no longer the modern view. Behavior is understood as a result of a combination of what the parents and child bring to the relationship (Chess, Fernandez, and Korn, 1980). It is thus possible to have a normal child whose temperamental patterns do not match well with his parents' expectations or personalities. Understanding these patterns sometimes helps:

> When 6-year-old Alan started school, he cried and refused to communicate with his teacher or the other children. Cooperation in play and group activities was zero: he spent his time by himself. After two days of this his teacher and the principal recommended a mental health consultation for emotional disturbance. When the mother declined, she was seen as uncooperative at first. However, with the help of her family doctor she was able to convince the school staff that Alan would be fine if he was not forced and was given a little time; he had reacted this way before to major new situations. And she was right.

Children who react like Alan are sometimes referred to as "slow-to-warm-up." They take longer to adjust to changes and their reactions are more intense. An appreciation of this pattern leads to different ways of introducing change or to more patience in waiting for adjustment (Thomas and Chess, 1980).

Early Development

Chess (1978) and Thomas and Chess (1980) have described how children with rubella deafness were able to acquire language and to improve their level of functioning over a period of years. These researchers challenge the idea that there is only one way to develop: " . . . the assumption that the handicapped child's development must duplicate that of the nonhandicapped child, or else it is inferior, inevitably leads to self-fulfilling prophecies of actual inferior outcome" (Thomas and Chess, 1980, p. 28).

Greenberg (1980a, 1980b, and 1980c) has examined the behavior of preschool deaf children and their mothers. The Total Communication group showed less stress or pressure in the mothers and more relaxed communication. These mothers reported greater confidence and feelings of effectiveness, and their children showed better social development than those in an oral-only program.

Identification

Another important influence on children's development is *identification*: they adopt many of the characteristics, values, and mannerisms of their parents. For deaf children with hearing parents, it seems that the communication barrier can make identification difficult. Perhaps the children, knowing their parents are not like them in a major way, look elsewhere for their heroes. Whatever the reasons, deaf adults are needed to supplement what the hearing parents can do. This is why it is essential for the child to see deaf adults in positions of authority, performing capably. In addition to

their parents, deaf children need deaf heroes! Yet few
schools or early programs introduce deaf heroes; this is
unfortunate, for there are many. As a parent, you can help
to make your child proud of deaf people who deserve his
esteem (discussed further in Chapter 14).

Understanding the Feelings of Others

Through gradual separation and identification, children
become better able to care about others and to understand
their feelings. This is a slow process, in which communication
is very important. When your deaf child sees you with an
angry look on your face, or sees you crying, curiosity about
the cause needs to be satisfied, and the feeling should be
labeled. Does an argument between mother and father mean
you don't love each other any more? Is a divorce to be
expected? How can you stop loving someone? How can you
hate someone you love? Will you stop loving me someday?
These are the kinds of endless, difficult, but vital questions
a secure hearing child asks. Your deaf child must be able to
do the same! This is where the methods controversy is clearly
not just a question of the best system for formal education
in the school, or of how well your child will talk later. Your
child's questions demand heart-to-heart answers that only
you can give, and they should be given at the right time—
when your child asks, not years later.

Unhealthy Uses of Deafness

There is one common pattern that is a serious risk for deaf
children—what is sometimes called "trading on deafness."
This refers to the very human tendency to make the most
of one's situation. Pity or guilt may be used by the deaf child
to manipulate people. This may be the case with parents,
with grandparents, or with strangers.

One 14-year-old deaf boy visited banks and opened illegal bank accounts. He
had raffle tickets printed to non-existent events and sold them. This went on for
several years until his activities came to the attention of the police. When the
people who had indulged him were asked why they allowed themselves to be
duped, they typically answered . . . "I felt sorry for him." Applying the same
standards to him as to hearing teenagers either never occurred to them or would

have seemed cruel, but these attitudes, of which he was fully aware, allowed him to develop into a "confidence man."

Adolescence

The usual idea that adults have about adolescents is that they go through a period of confusion, unhappiness, rebellion, and emotional upheaval. Although this describes some teenagers, the concept of "emotional turmoil" as normal in adolescence has been rejected by recent research. It is true, however, that for many children with disabilities, adolescence poses special tasks.

> Richard, at 14, was moved from a residential school to a local high school on the recommendations of the educational staff. His parents liked the idea of having him live at home, which seemed especially reasonable since he had been well-adjusted. In spite of all efforts he found the intense social life of his peers impossible to enter. Although he got some recognition for his athletic ability, at parties or on dates he felt at a loss. The others were not cruel to him; he was simply by-passed. For the first time Richard and his parents had to face the fact that good academic performance and fairly good oral skills were not enough.

Adjustment to a disability by child and by family during childhood does not ensure that adolescence will be without difficulties. Teenagers feel differently about themselves and about their place in society. They need close friendships and good opportunities for communication. Social skills become more important, and deficiencies are judged more harshly by peers. A reassessment of your child's potentialities may pose a great adjustment task for you as well. This is a time when many parents can benefit from discussions with others or with knowledgeable counselors.

Behavior Problems

Almost all studies of behavior problems come to the same conclusion: children who are deaf are more likely than hearing children to show disorders of behavior (Denmark et al., 1979; Freeman, 1979; Meadow, 1980; Meadow and Trybus, 1979; Schlesinger, 1978b). Depending upon how a behavior disorder is defined, the comparison might be something like 7%–10% of hearing children with disorders and 20%–30% of deaf children. Some workers feel that children with the rubella syndrome are more likely to have psychiatric problems (Chess et al., 1971).

Deaf children with deaf parents seem to behave better. The reasons for these differences are complex and not fully understood; they are certainly not the same for all children. It is much easier to find factors or situations that are *associated* with behavior disorder than to prove they *cause* it. A few relevant factors include: broken homes, family strife, severe psychiatric disorder in mothers, frequent changes of schools, repeated hospitalizations in early life, and proven damage to the brain. For many deaf children with behavior problems, the "cause" seems to be related to a failure of socialization. This means that the children have not learned enough about what is expected of them and why, or about how to obtain satisfaction of their needs in approved ways.

Young children at age two or three often have temper outbursts when they do not get their own way. When they seem to lose all contact with their environment while this happens, the episode is referred to as a "tantrum." Children who are deaf are reported to have many outbursts and tantrums when they are frustrated, and these disruptions seem to continue on to an older age than is encountered in most hearing children. Again, deaf parents have little or none of this special difficulty with their deaf child. As the child acquires ways of verbalizing needs instead of acting physically, more control over behavior is achieved. There seems to be no reason to think that the process of overcoming temper is any different for children who are deaf, as long as parent and child can communicate well.

PROVIDING OPPORTUNITIES FOR LEARNING

Incidental Learning

Hearing children are sometimes described as "all ears": they listen in on private conversations and pick up all sorts of information and misinformation without trying. This is

called *incidental learning*, which just happens, without
planning. Just this type of incidental learning can be missed
by deaf children in a hearing family in which they cannot
"overhear" what is going on. Because this is so vital, it is
believed by Total Communication advocates that children
who are deaf need to "oversee" conversations. Otherwise
many situations are puzzling: Why is Mommy angry after
she talks with Dad? Is it my fault? Why did they decide not
to go shopping as they had planned to do? Hearing children
recognize the sequence of events effortlessly. Deaf children
can only do the same if their parents learn to sign and if
they use it even when they are not addressing their child.
(In practice this is not likely to be done 100% of the time,
but whatever can be done will help.)

Total Family Involvement

Learning only a few signs is not enough. The mother
learning to sign is fine, but this is not as helpful as when the
whole family learns. Mothers cannot act as perpetual interpreters for father, siblings, visitors, and television! The
results of *not* doing this are apparent at any meeting run by
hearing people where deaf persons are present. It is likely
that even with a competent interpreter, the hearing people
will talk among themselves and that several will speak at
once. Too much will happen to be grasped by the deaf
people unless all are aware of the need to transmit all
information through the interpreter. If the deaf persons ask
or say something that is not quite on the topic, you can
recognize that important information was not communicated
to them.

Planned Learning

Planned learning is also important. You can help your child
gain an understanding of the world of work through a visit
to your place of employment. Excursions to museums or
other points of interest are other examples of planned

learning experiences. A discussion of who is in your family and their relationships with each other is also helpful for many children. Pictures can be shown to the child as a stimulus for discussion. Participation in family responsibilities (shopping, paying bills, planning a meal) will broaden your child's knowledge.

Sex and Family Life Education

Sex education should start early with awareness of the body and its functions, and of the attitudes of parents toward these functions. Caley and Gibson (1978) point out that many deaf children and teenagers have so little useful knowledge in this area that they are at the mercy of their own feelings, their ignorance, and the misinformation of others. A useful communication system will assist the home and school in providing realistic facts about sex and an appreciation of responsibilities toward others.

Responsible sexual behavior depends upon caring about others. Attending to pets or taking some responsibility for younger children may help to convey the need for caring, but deaf children should have the same opportunities as hearing children to see their parents and siblings expressing affection and concern for each other.

SOCIAL RELATIONSHIPS

Importance of the Family

The family is the child's most important source of early learning about social relationships. The interactions they see, and the kind of respect they perceive among family members are likely to have a powerful and life-long influence.

Friendships

In the Vancouver study (Freeman et al., 1975), it was found that deaf children (all of whom were living at home) were found to be much less likely to have playmates their own age than were hearing children. The subject of friendships is a sensitive one that returns us to the *methods controversy*. The idea that your deaf child will be fully accepted by hearing children is a compelling one. Any parent is likely to be concerned if a child is not participating in play with neighborhood peers. At first, interaction may be possible for young deaf and hearing children, because at an early age verbal interchange is not so crucial. As the basis for friendships changes, however (well described by Selman and Selman, 1979), deaf children gradually tend to be excluded from play activities (Meadow, 1980). If you have doubts about this statement, visit (unobserved) an elementary school that has a class (oral-only or Total Communication) of deaf children of ages nine to twelve. See what happens at recess time, at lunch, or on the playground. Usually the children who are deaf stay together, despite all efforts to integrate them socially, and despite their facility with speech.

This is not a plea for enforced separation. If hearing children are willing to make the effort to communicate with and to understand deaf children, this is fine. However, these relationships cannot be made a basis for socialization. Your child will need *close* friends to share secrets with, to love, hate, reject, and forgive. Without easy communication this is unlikely to happen. Many parents find that it is necessary to bring their child together with another deaf peer, even if that means extra effort.

One of the disadvantages of educational *integration* or *mainstreaming* is that a regular class or a special class in an ordinary school is not likely to provide your child with a wide enough range of choices of friends. There is no reason why two or three deaf children should automatically like each other as close friends. (This subject is discussed in greater detail in Chapter 18.)

Development of Social Skills

Rejection of your child by hearing children may have nothing to do with deafness. Children are very sensitive to the social abilities of other children. If your child cannot share (when others can), if reactions to frustration are excessive, or if he or she must always be the leader or make the rules, then lasting or even brief friendships are unlikely. Tolerance of frustration seems especially valuable to deaf children, as is a sense of humor. No one knows exactly how to ensure that these good qualities are impressed, but starting early with good communication and opportunities for sharing seems sensible. Sports and other games are excellent ways to develop these skills.

Deaf parents may have a special task with their deaf child: teaching about non-verbal communication. For example, noises that deaf people make unconsciously may be offensive to hearing people. Deaf children need to learn about how their non-verbal communication affects others. Sometimes deaf parents are also unaware of these noises and the teaching must be done by others.

Dating

Most deaf teenagers will date others who are deaf. Each family has different values concerning the age when dating should be allowed to start, whether single dating or only group activities should be permitted, what are suitable hours for returning home, and how to view sexual behavior. The only comment appropriate here is that adolescents should be aware of their parents' values, whether they obey them or not. Most professionals who work with teenagers agree that abandoning adolescents to their peer group without any guidance is dangerous. Many adolescents want, at times, to resist strong peer-group pressures, but cannot do so on their own. Perhaps they will blame their parents for being "old-fashioned," but this may be far preferable to irresponsible behavior resulting from lack of guidance.

THE COMMUNITY

Neighbors and friends of the family may need education about your deaf child and about deafness. Some will be helpful, others may have attitudes you don't like and simply cannot change. Encountering a child who is "different" seems to bring out the best in some people and the worst in others. Strangers who ordinarily would not think of intruding may ask pertinent or impertinent questions or may offer strange pieces of advice. (After a few months most parents seem to develop a way to handle these unexpected encounters.)

The use of non-relatives as baby-sitters is advisable so that your child can get used to the idea of separation and also to the rules and ways of others. Naturally it will be necessary to select such a person with care and to do some explaining about how to communicate with your child. Responsible deaf teenagers make excellent baby-sitters because of the additional opportunity for easy communication.

Participation in some community activities (such as Boy Scouts) is probably good for all children. Because deaf children find it harder to learn incidentally, they may have an even greater need to learn about others in their community; but they may need interpreters and special assistance in order to benefit from these experiences.

SPECIAL SITUATIONS

Single-parent families are becoming more common in many countries. Usually it is the mother who has custody of the child. If there is no substitute partner involved, a greater burden falls on the parent and some of the deaf child's needs may not be met as easily. Sometimes relatives or friends can help. In some areas it is possible to arrange for a "big brother" or "big sister" through an existing organization for that purpose (although communication may be a problem). Groups of deaf people may be a resource in some communities. [This subject has been discussed recently by Robinson (1979).]

A sad situation for some families is the decision not to use their native language with their child because they have moved to an area where another language is used. In the Vancouver area, for example, 22% of our deaf children are in homes where English is not the first language (Freeman et al., 1975). These parents would like their child to absorb their cultural heritage, yet it may be too much to expect many deaf children to master two or three languages when it is a major task for them to acquire one. There is no easy answer to this dilemma.

At some point your child is likely to ask you "Why am I deaf?" or "Would you love me more if I were hearing?" It is wise to think about these questions before they are asked, so you will not be overwhelmed and will not give an impulsive answer that you may regret later. In considering how to answer such a question, it is often helpful to find out whether this is really what the child is asking. "What do you want to know?" and "What started you thinking about that?" are questions that can give you a clue as to what the concern is. Obtaining the child's view first may also help. Ultimately there may be no satisfactory reply, especially if the cause is unknown. Even if you do answer to the best of your ability, these questions may come up again at a different stage of mental development. Sometimes the question represents worries about social acceptance by peers or insecurity about being loved by family members who are not deaf. What is most important is to leave the impression that whether there are easy answers or not, it is acceptable to ask and discuss such questions.

WHEN YOU NEED MORE HELP

Sometimes problems concerning deafness may become too much to handle on your own. The best first step under these conditions is to clarify the problem to someone you trust who is not afraid to listen and who does not tend to give quick advice. This could be a friend, relative, physician, or teacher. Parent groups may offer ideas to improve your coping skills and emotional support. If this is not enough, you need to decide *who* has the problem. Is it the child? You? Your spouse? The family? In large centers it may be fairly easy to obtain an evaluation of the total situation from a family service association, mental health or guidance clinic, or from an interested family physician, pediatrician, psychiatrist, or psychologist. In many other smaller areas such services do not exist and one must make the best of whatever resources are available.

Deafness may or may not be directly involved in the problem. If it is, this may pose a problem because so few mental health professionals are knowledgeable about deafness. Meadow and Trybus (1979) have stated that "it is the universal agreement of professionals experienced in such work with deaf persons that knowledge, training, and experience specific to deafness are essential to the provision of adequate mental health services" (p. 401).

Sometimes a compromise can be arranged: a flexible mental health worker (social worker, psychologist, or psychiatrist) can consult with an expert in deafness. Direct work with disturbed deaf children is difficult with an interpreter. Sometimes enough can be done with the family and school without treating the child.

It is likely that many problems could be avoided if parents could have enough early assistance to feel rewarded in raising a deaf child, and if later difficulties could be resolved before they became overwhelming.

SUMMARY

1. To give child-rearing advice is hazardous at best; there is little proof that we know how to prevent later problems by raising children in any specific way.
2. Mothers are especially likely to be heavily burdened if responsibilities for a deaf child are not shared. Fathers tend to be left out of contacts with those who are helping the deaf child and this may cause an imbalance in understanding and attitudes.
3. Angry feelings toward your child are usually a normal response to frustration. Generally the same expectations and limits should be set for deaf children as for hearing children.
4. Brothers and sisters need attention, too, and may react to an excessive focus on your deaf child.
5. Relatives can be both an important source of support and a negative influence; their importance should be considered in an overall plan for the deaf child.
6. Gradual separation of you and your child is important for healthy development.
7. Deaf children are more likely to have behavior problems and to act impulsively rather than with reflection. However, this is not true of deaf children with deaf parents, who seem to benefit from early communication and from their parents' easy acceptance of deafness.
8. Deaf children need deaf adults, in addition to their own parents, as models or as persons with whom to identify.
9. Incidental or unplanned learning is essential and is best provided when the whole family uses a clear method of communication even when the child is not being addressed directly.
10. Sex and family life education should begin early and should involve an awareness of how people can care about each other, be affectionate, and accept responsibilities.

11.   Friendships change as children grow older.
      When children are young, speech interchange is
      less important. Hearing friendships tend to be
      lost as children grow older. The close friends
      needed will usually be deaf.
12.   Adolescents need parental guidance to resist
      certain peer pressures.
13.   Awareness of, and participation in the
      community are necessary.
14.   Some special situations are briefly discussed in
      the chapter, such as single-parent families, the
      use of other languages in the home, and
      questions asked by the child about deafness.
15.   Mental health or counseling needs are not easily
      met because of the specialized nature of
      deafness. Compromise arrangements can
      sometimes be made.

Chapter 14

DEAF CULTURE
Expanding Horizons
for the Deaf Child

Speaking as a deaf person I believe that the most effective "cure" for deafness
is not medicine, not mechanical or electronic devices nor the surgical blade, but
understanding. And, ironically, understanding is free. Before we can develop
understanding, however, we must create awareness. [Gannon, 1979]

. . . profound deafness is much more than a medical diagnosis: it is a cultural
phenomenon in which social, emotional, linguistic, and intellectual patterns and
problems are inextricably bound together. [Meadow, 1975, p. 16]

INTRODUCTION

In this chapter we will discuss how awareness and understanding (which Gannon defines as essential) can be developed in deaf children and their families. No doubt our ideas
are still very incomplete; much more useful experience needs
to be examined.

We first discuss some ideas about culture; then at the
end of the chapter we present an example of how a sense of
exciting life possibilities and believable history were communicated to a group of deaf children.

WHAT IS CULTURE?

The concept of *culture* is not immediately easy to grasp.
Sometimes it is used to mean the "best" or "highest" creative
productions of a society, such as its art, music, and literature.

189

In this chapter, we use the word "culture" in a broader sense than this. One of the best nineteenth century definitions is: "that complex whole which includes knowledge, belief, art, morals, law, custom, and any other capabilities and habits acquired by man as a member of society" (Tylor, 1871, p. 1). Culture enables us to read meaning into what other people do (Hall, 1973). We take culture for granted and are largely unaware of it; parts of it are observed by us only with great difficulty.

Culture is acquired *socially*, so language is an essential part of cultural development.

> Language is often one of the most important distinguishing features of a subgroup within a society. It can serve as a cohesive, defining source of pride and positive identification and simultaneously as a focus for stigma and ridicule from members of the majority culture. [Meadow, 1975, p. 17]

For our purposes it is essential to realize that the broad definition of culture used above says nothing about whether parts of it are to be considered "good" or "bad," desirable or undesirable. Jokes and graffiti, attitudes toward time (keeping appointments, maintaining traditional work hours, "wasting" time), eating habits, ways of showing or controlling emotions, and in-group jokes and folklore are all part of culture.

WHY IS CULTURE IMPORTANT?

The lack of understanding of other cultures has been a major source of trouble for mankind. Although culture provides us with a framework for action in daily life, it also limits us in many ways. Because it is so complex and is acquired over so long a period of time, we are largely unaware of it. It may make us rigid and unreasonable with people who are different. For example, the ways in which children are taught, the subjects that are considered impor-tant, and the way in which these subjects are interpreted are a part of each nation's culture, and these traits cannot be easily exported to another culture. Hall (1973) states that it seems "inconceivable to the average person brought up in one culture that something . . . basic . . . could be done any differently from the way they themselves were taught (p. 48). Just why we feel so complacent and smug can be explained only by the blindness that culture imposes on its members" (p. 49). When people start arguing about what is "natural," including language, culture is always involved. (This has happened frequently with sign languages.)

We believe that an appreciation of *deaf* culture is basic for the development of children who are deaf. In helping your child, you as the parent can best determine how to approach this broad area we have called culture.

IS THERE A "DEAF CULTURE"?

The answer to the question "Is there a 'deaf culture'?" is yes. A deaf person's awareness of and participation in deaf culture may vary considerably, however. We may be uncomfortable with the idea of our children belonging to a "different culture" from our own. It may seem to place an obstacle between parent and child, but we should not oversimplify.

Let's look for a moment at the position in society of a totally different group, such as soldiers. Isn't it true that they have a somewhat different outlook on life than civilians do, that they enjoy talking about different subjects, that there are different expectations for them? If this is true, then in a sense they have different cultural characteristics. Of course in other ways they are more or less a part of the culture of their neighborhood, country, and perhaps race, religion, or ethnic group. They may have much in common with soldiers of other countries, and together they may feel misunderstood or unappreciated by civilians and politicians, while at the same time they may feel a sense of pride in activities foreign to most people. (We could have chosen many other groups for this example: mountaineers, physicians, astronauts.)

In a somewhat similar way, differences in outlook and experience make many deaf persons feel part of a "community" without living in a separate area. It is misleading to talk of "choosing" *either* the "deaf world" (or "ghetto") *or* full integration into "the hearing world." Be skeptical if you hear or read of someone arguing in these absolute terms.

As Schowe (1979) stated well: ". . ., the average citizen, hearing or deaf, is a member of many . . . 'we-groups.' A duplication, or plurality, of loyalties is clearly implied. Membership in a 'we-group' does not isolate anyone from membership in a variety of other 'we-groups'" (p. 42). Schowe knows what he is talking about; he has been part of several "we-groups." Born with progressive deafness, he graduated from Gallaudet College in 1918, then worked as a labor economics specialist for the Firestone Tire and Rubber Company. His deaf son is an educator of the deaf with a Ph.D. degree. In Schowe's book (written at age 86), he concludes: "In my own view, the deaf society is of prime importance. It is in the milieu of this social structure that the deaf gain a self-respecting image of themselves and a productive relationship with others" (p. 37).

On the other hand, some people ignore deaf culture altogether, or see it as something totally negative. For example, Knox (1976), who works in an oral-only program, gives many good ideas about working with parents in groups. She shows compassion and insight, but she does not say one word about deaf adults or their culture.

Sometimes you may see the term "subculture" used, to refer to a linguistic community with a larger culture surrounding it. Although this term does apply to deaf people, we will not use it because of the negative connotations that a subculture is something inferior.

Feeling comfortable with other people's way of life is not easy. Deaf culture and language have suffered from neglect and outright persecution, but attitudes are changing toward those deaf persons who are not afraid to show that they are deaf. A few examples of changes and contrasts follow.

At a meeting in 1975 a leading educator of the deaf from a European country recounted two anecdotes: 1) two deaf women she knew boarded a bus on which she was a passenger and refused to sign to her or to each other because they were ashamed to do so in public; 2) in her country deaf children were separated in schools by sex, and the boys and girls actually had rather different sign languages; how they were supposed to relate to each other was not at all clear.

In the United States, where signing in schools was forbidden (by law in at least one state), children who were caught at it were made to sit on their hands or were otherwise humiliated. Now signing is becoming more prominent on television. The news is interpreted, presidential candidates learn a few signs, people who use signs are shown on adult and children's TV without ridiculing them for not speaking well; this is part of a greater and healthier acceptance of alternative life-styles. (Deaf people were amused that the first TV advertisement to be interpreted for them was for a well-known laxative!)

Few hearing people take the trouble to try to understand why deaf persons need a sense of community among themselves. This neglect is not deliberately malicious, but it is more than ignorance. It comes from ingrained patterns of thinking that the way the majority does things (including communicating) is just "naturally" right (Cicourel and Boese, 1972). Unfortunately, many of those who make important decisions for deaf children also think this way. You, yourself, will have to take time to gradually feel your way into deaf culture. It will require a restructuring of your presumptions about how to understand the world.

WHY IS THERE A DEAF CULTURE?

Deaf people see the world differently in some respects because their lives are different. "As deaf children mature, they do not find satisfactory role models within their family" (Schein, 1979b, p. 48). The minority-group situation in which this places them is unusual (Meadow, 1980; Vernon and Makowsky, 1969). They may be deprived of certain cultural and linguistic opportunities because their status as a minority group is unclear to most people. This may result in more of a handicap than deafness itself (Jacobs, 1974). Deaf people's needs are likely to be overlooked because those making decisions for them only have a second-hand knowledge of what it is like to be deaf.

Hearing families who sign need to provide broad cultural, social, and linguistic contacts for their deaf child (as do deaf parents for their hearing children).

There are more obvious reasons for the existence of deaf culture. Deaf people can generally enjoy each other's company because communication is not a problem and because of shared life experiences. Deaf organizations include hundreds of clubs, sports events (including international games), their own insurance company (because of rate discrimination in the past), and dance and theater groups of professional quality. These would not exist if they were not meeting a real need.

ETHNOCENTRISM

Ethnocentrism refers to the tendency to place our own experiences, values, and attitudes in a central position, viewing those of others as strange and inferior. If hearing persons regard the way deaf people communicate (using their hands, voice, facial expression, and space) as naturally inferior, then they will convey a sense of rejection and condescension that may be damaging to a deaf child.

Language and sense of self are intertwined. There have been many attempts to stamp out a culture through eliminating its language (Farb, 1974). As applied to deafness, for example, Dr. Leo Connor, Executive Director of the Lexington School for the Deaf (a well-known oral school in New York City), stated:

Educators, parents, and deaf children must be assured of the most important fact of all concerning the minority group of the deaf: that a handicapped person is like everyone else and that his own and the majority's viewpoint of his handicap fundamentally agree. . . . *We should hope and work for the day when there is no subculture of the deaf* . . . anything less than commitment to total integration into a hearing society is a goal that cannot be acceptable to parents of deaf children. [Connor, 1972, pp. 524–525, emphasis added]

This kind of approach almost never succeeds, and it tends to produce undesirable effects: resentment, and even resistance to learning or to using the language of "the oppressors." The language of deaf people has been largely an "underground" language until recently. Deaf adults who lived through these times tell us how they associated sign language with secrecy, inferiority, and sometimes the smell of urine (because the only safe place to sign in school was in the lavatory).

Ethnocentrism is a common tendency that we all must struggle against if we are to achieve true tolerance and acceptance of human differences. In doing this we must be cautious about the opposite effect: creating false pride in deaf children so that they ignore or look down upon other cultures (including the majority language). This attitude is as undesirable as the suppression of deaf culture.

DEAF HERITAGE

There has been a significant increase in the attention paid to deaf heritage in recent years. An important book on this subject by Jack Gannon of Gallaudet College is being published to coincide with the Centennial of the National Association of the Deaf in 1980. Calendars with stories of famous deaf Americans will be an annual feature. In fact, there is too much happening to summarize it all here. Your family, your deaf child, and you will find these developments of interest. In a 1979 speech, Jack Gannon pointed out some little-known things that deaf people have done, such as founding over 40 American schools for the deaf, flying a light plane solo across the United States in 1947, editing more than a dozen newspapers, inventing a well-known shorthand method, and founding the Girl Scouts of America.

It is important for all deaf children to be informed about deaf culture and about future possibilities for people who are deaf. Without special efforts from their families and schools, it may be difficult for deaf children to feel that it is "OK" to be deaf.

When parents and children both share the same cultural identity, patterns are usually transmitted effortlessly as a part of daily life. However, if deaf parents were made to feel that it is bad to be deaf, their children are likely to acquire the same negative attitudes. You may therefore meet deaf people who are ashamed of being deaf, of signing, or of their poor English. This low self-image may be the result of the misguided efforts of parents and schools to create, out of a deaf person, the facsimile of a hearing person.

BILINGUALISM AND BICULTURALISM

Bilingualism is the use of two languages; biculturalism is the existence or encouragement of two cultural patterns. We believe both are appropriate for deaf persons. Although bilingualism is taken for granted in many parts of the world where it has obvious practical value, it has been mistrusted and discouraged in North America and in Britain. Only recently has there been an American thrust toward reviving pride in (and usage of) different languages and cultures rather than advocating the "melting pot" philosophy. A "Bilingual Education Act" (P.L. 90–247, Title VII, ESEA) was passed in 1968. Included in the concept of bilingual education is the study of the history and culture that are associated with the mother tongues. The program is intended to develop and maintain children's self-esteem and pride in both their native and American cultures. Canada has attempted not only to foster French and English bilingualism, but also to preserve (rather than to absorb) the culture of its citizens who come from many lands.

Although deaf children need pride in deaf people's accomplishments, they also need a good working knowledge of the language and culture of the majority if they are to take successful advantage of all that life has to offer. This implies that parents and schools need to teach life skills and to help deaf children understand how social relationships are initiated and maintained.

THE CENTRALIZED SCHOOL AS A FOCUS OF DEAF CULTURE

For many years schools for the deaf (especially residential schools) have been focuses of deaf culture. It was largely in residential schools that deaf people learned about life from each other, and deaf children from hearing families encountered fluent signing.

For the purposes of this discussion we are talking about children who need signing, and who cannot function fully in an oral-only situation. In a school for the deaf (day or residential) there is a sufficient number of children to justify the following: staff, *all* of whom (not just teachers) can communicate with the children; auditory and audiovisual equipment; teams, clubs, dances, and parties; models of adult deaf leadership and language; and possibilities for leadership by the child within the total school. These children can truly "belong." There is no easy way to match these advantages for deaf children in a self-contained special class or in a regular class in a hearing school. The *quality* of centralized schools is not the question here. Some day schools or residential schools may be inadequate in most or all of the areas of importance that we have identified. However, to abandon the centralized school or to restrict it to those deaf children who are multiply handicapped, emotionally disturbed, or who have failed in other settings would be tragic and illogical. Yet it is happening now. Accusations have been made of "racism" and "cultural genocide." These may seem extreme terms to apply, but if the centralized facilities cease to exist, much of value may be irretrievably lost.

We need to recognize the social, linguistic, and cultural facts and to adapt them to the most appropriate educational setting for each child. Even poor residential schools have graduated deaf students who are socially, emotionally, and academically well developed. This is something that educators did not plan. If the option to attend a special school is taken away in favor of mainstreaming and "improving" education, the damage to deaf culture may take decades to reverse.

There is always room for improvement in any educational program and this also is true for centralized schools. Changes require understanding, wisdom, support from educational authorities, and the participation of parents, and deaf children and deaf adults in working out a logical plan. Otherwise the way the schools function will be a combination of personalities, luck, and expediency. They may still offer much that is positive, although not by design. Their potential for excellence will not be realized. This is more a matter of attitudes than of money.

SPECIFIC SUGGESTIONS FOR
INVOLVEMENT IN DEAF CULTURE

1. Learn about deaf people and their accomplishments. A good start would be the book *Notable Deaf Persons* by Braddock and Crammatte (1975) and a subscription to *Gallaudet Today.* (The latter has many items of international interest.) *FOCUS,* a publication of the National Technical Institute for the Deaf, is available free from their Public Information Office. Publications of your local or national organizations of or for deaf people are also appropriate (such as *The Endeavor* of the IAPD, *Hearing* of the RNID, the *Deaf American* and *Deaf Canadian,* the *British Deaf News,* and the Newsletter of the National Union of the Deaf). Learn all you can about deaf people in your area and tell your child stories about their accomplishments. When older, your child may appreciate poetry by deaf poets, such as that of Miles (1976) and Smith (1973).

2. Bring deaf people into contact with your child, as friends (if that is possible), as house guests, or as baby-sitters. Invite other deaf children to visit or to stay overnight as company for your child. Learn first-hand some of the special ways deaf people have developed to get along in situations like ordering in a restaurant, fielding comments from strangers, and signing in public. You may need some assistance when first making contacts.

3. After you become familiar with some deaf people, visit deaf clubs, churches, conventions, sports events, and the like. You will then find ways to share with your child these areas of life as a deaf person. (Again, this does not mean plunging into a deaf activity without some knowledge of sign language and a guide, who might be a more experienced parent or a deaf person who can communicate with you.)

4. Insist that your school or preschool hire qualified deaf teachers and professionals, that it make every reasonable effort to include deaf persons in its various activities, and that it encourage cultural events (deaf speakers at graduation ceremonies, for example). Although culture cannot be taught as such, teachers should have training in deaf studies; even teachers who are deaf may profit from attention to this topic.

5. Join a parent organization and the IAPD (see address in back of this book). Encourage your group to invite deaf speakers and to organize panel presentations and discussions by deaf adults and teenagers.

6. Have deaf speakers discuss career preparation. Visit deaf workers on the job with your child.

7. Get book lists (such as those of the IAPD, National Association of the Deaf, British Deaf Association, and Gallaudet College; we have listed some others in the back of this book). In particular, obtain books or materials about deaf persons for your child.

8. Improve your sign language. Don't be satisfied if you can "get by" with your child, because it can be misleading. Try to have some regular exposure to situations where you must communicate with different deaf persons.

9. Install doorbell lights and save money to purchase a TDD (see Chapter 20). This will open access to your home for deaf people and will let your child easily contact deaf friends.

This does not mean giving up all your other interests and activities. It may not be easy to tell whether you are "doing enough." Some people may tell you that you are not, no matter how hard you try. Others may provide reassurance when you yourself are convinced that you are slacking. If you can sense gradual improvement in your skills and understanding, if you get pleasure from knowing deaf people, if you see signs of pride in your deaf child, and if you feel you are enjoying life, then you are probably doing well. A change of attitude toward deafness is what is likely to help. All these suggestions are ways of assisting your family toward participation in deaf culture; they are not rules to be slavishly followed.

A SHORT STORY ABOUT A WONDERFUL DEAF MAN

The following talk, given by Jack Gannon to the graduating students of the Kendall Demonstration Elementary School for the Deaf in Washington, D.C. on June 17th, 1975, is reprinted here by permission. It is an example of a topic in deaf studies.

This morning I would like to tell you a story about a very wonderful deaf man. This man had a lot of ambition. He not only dreamed about many important things but he knew that with hard work he could make his dreams come true.

He is a very smart man and he knows so many big words that they can choke a typewriter. He has always worked with such drive and enthusiasm that you would think his pants were on fire.

This man is tall and thin and he has wavy hair. There is always a grin on his face and a twinkle in his eyes. He is a man who lives by the motto "Do it NOW!"

This man, let's call him David, was born in 1900 in Yanoschina, a small village in southern Russia. He had nine brothers and sisters.

One day when he was five years old he decided he was old enough to go to school. So one cold winter morning without his mother's or sisters' knowledge he followed his older sisters to school. In those days there were no buses and children had to walk long distances to school. It was very cold that morning and it began snowing very hard. His sisters walked very fast and he couldn't keep up with them. Soon he became lost and he got very tired and sat down in the snow to rest.

Later that morning David's mother noticed that he was missing. Quickly she called on neighbors and friends to help her search for David. When they found him he was very cold and had almost frozen to death. He was sick for a long time afterwards, but he lived. That is how he became deaf.

When David was six years old his family moved to Canada and he entered the Manitoba School for the Deaf. He was a smart young man and soon became bored with school and quit. His father sent him to a linotype school where he became a printer. One day a wise old deaf printer took young David aside and said: "You are a very smart boy. You are wasting your brains here. Go to college!" David was surprised. He had never heard of a college for deaf students. From this wise old deaf man he learned about Gallaudet College and decided to enter.

When David graduated from Gallaudet College he realized how fortunate he had been and decided to go back to Canada and help deaf people there. He founded the Canadian Association of the Deaf and raised $50,000 to send deaf students to college. He founded the *OAD News*, a newspaper for the deaf in Canada. He became active in many organizations of the deaf. Later he helped the Gallaudet College Alumni Association raise money for its Centennial Fund.

What made this man so successful? Many things. He has a wonderful wife and two daughters who always encouraged him. He was a smart man and he was not afraid of hard work. He was a man who would never accept "no" or "can't" for an answer. To those words he had a response. "Bunk," he would say, meaning *nonsense*, or in his language meaning: "let's not waste time; let's do it NOW!"

In 1970 that man retired from his job at Gallaudet College. He has received many, many honors because people appreciate his hard work and what he did for deaf people.

A few years ago the man I am talking about suffered a stroke. It paralyzed part of his side and made communicating very difficult for him. But he's a very stubborn man and after about six months' illness he was up and about again. He is now 75 years old and he volunteers his time to work at Gallaudet College.

This is a very short story about a man named Dr. David Peikoff. He is here today and I want you to meet him. He did not know I was going to talk about him.

This story is about only one successful deaf person. There are thousands and thousands of other success stories like this one. Look around you at Dr. Davila, at your deaf teachers and counselors. They have succeeded and become productive citizens. If hard work does not bother you, you can succeed too. Perhaps some day I will have the privilege to tell some school children a story about YOU. Good luck and God bless you.

DISCUSSION AND CONCLUSIONS

The concepts of deaf culture and studies are sometimes misunderstood. We are stressing bilingual, bicultural considerations because they are often neglected (as is evident when looking at current books on deafness). Amplification, auditory training, speech, reading, sign languages, signing codes, and deaf culture are *all* important. Choosing one of them does not exclude any other.

No claim is being made that introducing deaf culture will solve all problems. It has never been systematically explored. Our recommendations are based upon new understandings of the social usage of language (sociolinguistics)

(Trudgill, 1974), the recent work on sign languages reviewed in Chapter 11, the good adjustment and performance of deaf children who have deaf parents, and our better understanding of how life is lived by deaf adults (Higgins, 1980; Jacobs, 1974).

The inclusion of deaf culture should not mean that other cultural influences are ignored: remember that we are all members of many "we-groups." Parents and educators should take the implications of culture seriously. If we want deaf children to feel good about themselves by realizing what deaf people have done and can do, we should do everything we can to *integrate* cultural experiences. We have suggested some of the ways in which this might be done by parents and schools, but these are certainly not the only ways.

We hope that those involved with deafness begin to see that pride and confidence may be boosted by taking advantage of cultural opportunities. Cultural experiences are valuable in their own right—just as important for development as amplification, caring parents, and devoted teachers of academic subjects. It is *not* an either/or question.

The so-called missionary spirit is not appropriate with deaf people. Years ago, North American and European missionaries traveled to far-off lands. There they preached their religion and introduced some of the benefits of Western health care, but they also *imposed* their culture by designating how the "natives" should dress and work, and by specifying even the details of their ceremonies and sexual behavior. All of this dominance depended upon the missionaries' assumption of superiority. Many professionals have treated deaf people in the same overpowering and inappropriate way.

If it should be argued that integration into deaf culture is too radical because there is insufficient evidence for effectiveness, we would counter by saying: 1) until the method is tried, there can be no adequate evaluation; and 2) the restrictive oral-only system that dominated the field of education of the deaf and the lives of deaf adults for a century was based upon *no* scientific evidence of success. We favor change *and* evaluation of results.

Imagine that a school principal and his or her staff met regularly with deaf people (children and adults) and parents to discuss and implement the components of deaf culture and deaf studies in the school program (academic and extra-curricular). Suppose they did this sincerely, out of conviction that it needed to be done. The changes could be amazing. Deaf children and adults could begin to feel that it is "OK" to be deaf, that they are as good as anyone else, and that their ideas are being considered and sometimes actually are being put into practice. Relations with the deaf community would greatly improve. The process could be monitored and evaluated; there are investigators who would love to do this. Could this ever be more than just a dream?

SUMMARY

1. Culture refers to the ways, customs, and attitudes
    of a group of persons; it is largely unconscious,
    transmitted through language, and overlaps other
    sets of attitudes.
2. A culture is not "good" or "bad" in itself, nor
    does culture consist only of "the finer things."
3. Deaf people have a culture that has been
    misunderstood and persecuted for almost 100
    years.
4. Although there is a "culture of schools" (Chapter
    18), deaf culture in schools has not been given a
    place of significance.
5. Hearing families who are unfamiliar with deafness
    cannot themselves provide enough "culture" for
    their child. A number of suggestions have been
    given for enhancing the child's sense that it is
    acceptable to be deaf and that deaf people can
    accomplish much. Suggestions include providing
    contacts with other deaf persons and encouraging
    bilingualism and biculturalism at home and at
    school.
6. Once deaf culture and language are accepted as
    being equal to others, there are beneficial
    consequences: respect from hearing persons, a
    greater sense of dignity and self-worth for deaf
    children, better acceptance by them of the
    language and culture of the majority, and the
    development of creative ways of using culture for
    the good of all persons.

Chapter 15

EARLY INTERVENTION PROGRAMS

The evidence indicates that the family is the most effective and economical system for fostering and sustaining the development of the child. The evidence indicates further that the involvement of the child's family as an active participant is critical to the success of any intervention program. [Bronfenbrenner, 1976, pp. 251–252]

. . . children of hearing parents . . . have more preschool experience and tutoring and come from families with higher socioeconomic levels and more standard English patterns. Yet the children of deaf parents exhibit educational, social, and communicative superiority. One can only speculate on the attainments of deaf children of hearing parents if—in addition to familial, social, educational, and economic advantages—they had benefited from some form of early systematic communication with their parents. [Moores, 1978b, p. 180]

INTRODUCTION

Deaf children who have deaf parents have an advantage that continues to increase into the adolescent years (Moores, Weiss, and Goodwin, 1981, in press). This observation has increased interest in deaf children. The research of Corson (1976) suggests that it is not only early communication, but also easier and better acceptance of their children by deaf parents that may be involved (children of deaf parents who used speech and gestures instead of signing were still superior to those of hearing parents).

We have not yet discussed specific types of programs for deaf children and their families, but in the next chapters we apply the general principles outlined previously. Because there are many different ways to assist young deaf children and their families, we divide the chapters by age ranges. This chapter focuses on children from birth to age three, by which time children should be ready for preschool (discussed in Chapter 16). After a presentation of learning vacations in Chapter 17, we discuss elementary and secondary schools in Chapter 18.

The most complete review of early intervention from the Total Communication viewpoint is by Moores (1978b). He points out that the terms used are confusing: "early intervention" may be used synonymously with (or sometimes distinguished from) "infant programs," "nursery programs," and "pre-preschool programs." Although he refers to all services prior to age 6 as "early intervention," we will preserve the age distinction mentioned above.

HISTORY

According to Moores (1978b), almost every component of a "new" or "innovative" program is in fact over 100 years old. These already existent components include the concept of integration, the early use of signs or fingerspelling, the teaching of signs to the hearing children in the program, total family involvement, home visits, and the use of residual hearing (although previously the technical means to enhance residual hearing were lacking).

Leaders in the field of deafness in the nineteenth century were aware of many of the same needs that we discuss here. In the past, most deaf children received little or no special help, unless the family was wealthy and could afford private tutoring.

The concepts mentioned above were "re-discovered" in the past 10 years. When teachers of the deaf started playing a larger role in the development of deaf babies, they were put in the difficult position of accepting the "responsibilities of parent counselors, social workers, child development specialists, educational audiologists, and psychologists—roles for which they were completely unqualified" (Moores, 1978b, p. 195).

Until recently only one early intervention approach that included manual communication had been used with deaf babies in North America: the Rochester Method in Rochester, New York. This remained the situation until the shift to Total Communication in the United States in the late 1960s (Moores, 1978b).

Only major cities in the developed countries had early services for deaf children. Many parents received no early services at all, except for amplification and advice to "talk, talk, talk." Most parents depended upon the correspondence course of the John Tracy Clinic in Los Angeles (founded 1943) until their child entered school at age five or six. (This course is free to parents of preschool-age deaf children.) By 1970 the course had served parents in 114 countries and was printed in 16 languages. Parents could write to the Clinic staff and receive individualized replies. (This was and is a purely oral program. There is at present no similar course for the Total Communication approach, except one for deaf-blind children provided by the Tracy Clinic.)

There seem to be five main reasons for the recent expansion of early intervention services: 1) dissatisfaction with results of the education of deaf children and an expectation that an earlier start would be better; 2) the concept of an "optimal period" for early language acquisition; 3) the general movement toward compensatory education for deprived, poor, or handicapped children, such as the Head Start programs in the United States; 4) technical advances in early screening, in early identification of deafness, in amplification, and in training of audiologists; and 5) the rubella epidemic of 1964–65 (the worst on record in North America), which necessitated the establishment of clinics and services because of increased numbers of deaf and multiply handicapped deaf children.

HOW EFFECTIVE ARE EARLY
INTERVENTION PROGRAMS?

Not many studies of the effectiveness of early intervention have been made. The evidence reviewed earlier in this book and the research of Mindel and Vernon in 1971 show that oral-only programs have not been very effective when compared to the accomplishments of deaf children with deaf parents. This is not the same, however, as demonstrating that an early intervention Total Communication program is better for deaf children of hearing parents than the oral-only approach. Recently Greenberg (1980a, 1980b, and 1980c) has shown the general superiority of Total Communication over oral-only programs with young children in terms of extended conversations and ease in relating with their mothers. An earlier start was associated with better results, but there are as yet no good *long-term* follow-up studies that tell us which parts of a program are essential for which children, and which components could be abandoned.

Soviet follow-up studies report substantial language gains in children who used what they term *neo-oralism*, or fingerspelling and speech (similar to the Rochester Method). (The quality of this research is in doubt, according to a personal communication from Moores, 1980.) The Russians had been disappointed with oral-only results. Fingerspelling with simultaneous speech is now the official approach used with young deaf children in Russia. Quigley (1969) confirmed the Russian experience in a comparative study in the United States. He found the Rochester Method children superior to oral-only children in written English, reading, and speechreading.

Although everyone seems to believe in it, the value and long-term effects of early intervention are yet to be convincingly demonstrated. In fairness, we should explain that it is very difficult (perhaps impossible) to do a truly *experimental* study that would prove, once and for all, the effectiveness of a particular type of program. Comparing different programs with children already assigned to them has its limitations—it can always be claimed that there were differences in the children from the start. In the ideal experimental study, one would randomly (that is, by chance) assign children to different groups, and suspend all clinical judgment or preferences. The parents could not have any say about the choice. Few parents would accept these unethical conditions!

WHAT DO PARENTS NEED?

No two families are the same; therefore, individual differences must be considered. After a diagnosis of deafness is made, and before a child is ready for preschool, family needs can be summarized as follows:

1. Repeated opportunity to ask questions and to learn about deafness, hearing aids, controversial issues, and language development.
2. Attention to family emotional needs (personal reaction to deafness, grief responses, marital problems).
3. Realization that families are not alone; others have also had problems with deafness, and have learned to cope with obstacles successfully (helpful activities include contact with other parents, group discussions, and learning about services that will be useful for their child) (IAPD, 1976).
4. Guided contact with deaf people (children and adults) to change ignorant and stereotypic ideas about deafness; appreciation of their language, modes of communication, and culture.
5. Assistance in answering the questions of the child's siblings and relatives, and enlistment of their support.
6. Learning to distinguish normal (but worrisome) patterns of behavior from those really caused by reactions to deafness; feedback on the question, "How am I doing as a parent?"
7. Support in learning to establish rewarding communication between child and family, rather than focusing on the mechanics of communication (especially the mechanics of speech).
8. Identification of any special situations that might affect the

deaf child's progress, and assistance in modifying them if
necessary.

9. Learning to have fun with their child.
10. A direct, home-based program to provide the most
    important of these components.
11. A dependable, compassionate professional who accepts and
    respects deaf people, and whom the parents like.

WHAT DOES THE CHILD NEED?

The child's needs are:

1. To be loved as a child first (not because of, or in spite of,
    deafness).
2. Involvement of the whole family in communication (IAPD,
    1976).
3. Models to identify with inside and outside of the family
    (Nordén, 1978).
4. To know that he or she is not the only deaf person in the
    world, to meet a wide variety of deaf people, and to feel
    part of a "respected minority group" (Nordén, 1978, p. 2).
5. A teacher to set up and monitor a home-based program that
    includes all useful means of communication and that
    promotes development of *all* communication and language
    skills.
6. Periodic re-evaluation, including evaluation of vision.

HOW ARE THE NEEDS OF
FAMILY AND CHILD TO BE MET?

Services to meet family and child needs ideally should be
available to *all* family members so that the mother does not
become the sole "expert" and communication go-between.
No one person will have all the necessary knowledge and
skills in deafness, child development, audiology, communication, and parent counseling. Several professionals' skills
will be needed, and these should be coordinated. The teacher
of the deaf may have the most opportunity to become aware

of problems requiring counseling, yet may have no training in this area, while those who have the skills may not have the contact with and trust of the family. (A consultant to the teacher can be helpful with problems that arise, and may not need to be involved directly.) It is very important that the teacher have experience with babies (including deaf babies) and preschool children. (A good indicator of the teacher's attitude toward deafness as a difference rather than a defect is to ask whether he or she has any deaf friends.)

AN EXAMPLE OF AN EARLY INTERVENTION PROGRAM

Because we believe our program in Vancouver has some unusual features that are consistent with the concepts presented in this book, we briefly describe it here (Carbin, 1976), but this should not be taken as a claim that we are entirely satisfied. An independent evaluation of our Counselling and Home Training Program for Deaf Children and Their Families will be completed in 1981. We hope it will fill some of the gaps identified earlier in assessing the effectiveness of early intervention programs.

Common Features

We share the following common features with many early intervention services (including oral-only): 1) information for parents, 2) early use of amplification, 3) audiologic re-assessments, 4) regular home visits by a teacher of the deaf, 5) periodic re-evaluation and discussion of progress with the parents, 6) involvement of the family, and 7) group sessions with parents.

Unusual Features

Our program also has some unusual features. We are fortunate to have early contact with parents and children, although often the diagnosis is later than we would like. Our program is based in the same location as that of the team making the diagnosis for most deaf children in British Columbia (the Children's Hospital Diagnostic Centre). If they wish to, parents can meet the program staff during the initial hearing assessment, which reduces further delay. The program staff has easy access to the team pediatrician, psychiatrist, otologist, neurologist, audiologist, nurse, psychologist, and social worker.

Parents are immediately informed about the oral-manual controversy and are encouraged, as a matter of policy, to visit both the oral program in the city and our Total Communication program to aid in making their own choice.

For those persons enrolled in our Program, emphasis is placed on total family involvement. Important relatives are included in counseling (when needed) and in weekly Parent Night group activities, including sign language instruction. Weekly visits by deaf adults and by a teacher of the deaf are arranged, insofar as possible, when other family members can also be present.

The Program has both a secretary-interpreter for the deaf director and a sociolinguistic consultant. Deaf children of deaf parents are also served, although their needs are somewhat different. Limited consultation services are offered to people from other parts of the Province; it is hoped that these services will be expanded soon.

Unique Features

We believe that there are several unique components to our program:

1. *Deaf director.* Parents, children, staff, and government need to communicate with a deaf person who is in a high-profile, professional position. (This helps to avoid the all-too-frequent delay by parents in meeting deaf people.) The director drives a car, has a sense of humor, and performs competently: in short, he is a person who happens to be deaf and is not miserable about it. Through the example of the director, parents can see possibilities for their own child,

but they can also recognize real limitations in spite of good speech and speechreading skills (the director became deaf at age four). The Children's Hospital and the Federal Government have made a commitment to this kind of organization, otherwise it would have been impossible to support (there are extra costs for an interpreter and for telecommunication devices).

2. *Use of prelingually deaf native signers.* A deaf adult visits each family on a regular basis, serving as a role and language model for the deaf child and for the parents. The child sees someone "deaf like me" who is a person of importance. The parents can then interact with a deaf individual who is different from the deaf director. They learn to communicate and to gain an expanding appreciation of life as a deaf person and of deaf culture. Later, a different deaf adult is assigned to the family so they encounter a variety of sign language "accents," auditory/oral abilities, life experiences, and personal styles.

   At weekly Parent Night meetings, all sign instructors are deaf adults. The overall role of deaf adults in the Program contrasts with the usual practice in the past. Previously, deaf teachers were forbidden to teach young deaf children unless the children were multiply handicapped, and hearing parents usually had little or no contact with deaf adults (Moores, 1978b).

3. *Deaf culture.* Although culture is emphasized by the participation of deaf adults as described above, there are other areas of importance. Deaf people are invited speakers at Parent Nights. Deaf leaders are invited to visit our program. Periodic picnics are organized with attendance by deaf staff and deaf parents. Another recent feature is the Learning Vacation Program, to be described in more detail in Chapter 17. It is helpful for hearing parents to see deaf people functioning as parents to their own children.

4. *Home visits by other staff.* The home may be visited by other workers (such as the child psychiatrist). This assists the professional in understanding how the family functions in its own natural setting, rather than in the artificial one of a clinic or office.

5. *Flexibility in sign usage.* No manually coded English system is prescribed. Most hearing parents use PSE (Pidgin Sign

English), moving toward the ASL end of the language spectrum when conversing with native signers (once they have enough experience) and toward the English end when that is appropriate. If parents wish to learn some parts of a manual English code such as Signed English, we have no objection. Frequent correction of the child's speech or signing is not encouraged. All parents learn to appreciate ASL as a valid, expressive language. The general approach could be termed *bilingual and bicultural*.

THE CHILD WITH MULTIPLE DISABILITIES

Although we deal with the complicated subject of multiple disabilities in Chapter 22, something should be said about it here. Because of the infinite variety of combinations of disabilities, no program can be designed around only one or two of them. Our own program was initially intended to serve deaf children without other disabilities, but that soon proved impossible. In fact, we have accepted deaf children with such additional labels of impairment as mental retardation, blindness, cerebral palsy, cleft palate, and autism. It is not easy for staff to work with some of these children without very specialized experience and training. We have combined our efforts with those of other agencies serving these disabilities, because there simply was no other place for the parents to go. Some children have progressed well, others have made only very slow gains.

Certain combinations of disabilities, such as hearing and visual impairment, may multiply problems rather than just adding their individual effects. This means that more complex techniques are needed than simply those a teacher of the deaf would use in combination with those suitable for the blind.

We are certainly not suggesting that programs for deaf children should exclude those children with additional impairments. What is essential is to assess whether these other impairments have any real consequences, as pointed out in Chapter 7. The label for the impairment is, in itself, not very helpful. Combining forces with other experienced workers is often necessary, although it must be recognized that more time will frequently be needed for this inter-agency cooperation to achieve results. Inclusion of multiply handicapped deaf children is easier in a home-based early intervention program than later in a preschool setting where children spend much of their time in a group. Some deaf children with multiple disabilities remain in our Counselling and Home Training Program until a later age, because they are not yet ready for preschool, at the usual age of about three.

CONCLUSIONS

Although proof of the benefits of early intervention programs is only now becoming available, there seems to be general agreement that deaf children with hearing parents do better when the diagnosis is early and when there is time to assist the family in accepting the child's deafness and in developing easy communication.

Assistance should include information (repeated as often as necessary), the opportunity to ask questions, support through the emotional crisis surrounding the diagnosis, hearing aids and instruction on their use and maintenance, feedback on child-rearing skills as applied to the deaf child, help in interpreting the meaning of deafness to relatives, and experiences with a wide variety of deaf persons (children and adults).

All of this assistance needs to be done in such a way as to encourage, rather than discourage, the active involvement of fathers, and to recapture satisfaction in family life. The aim is to create the favorable circumstances that are obtained when both parents are deaf: acceptance of the child and enjoyable communication. The *forms* of communication are less important than the *fact* of communication. Deaf children should be exposed to several language models. By the time they reach preschool, they should be able to communicate easily with deaf native signers and with their parents and teachers. They should be curious about the world and about English. True bilingualism is the goal. Speech and speech-reading skills are valued, but are not the measure of success.

Ideally, by the time their child reaches preschool age, parents should have acquired enough balance in their feelings and attitudes so that they can emotionally accept their child's deafness and can avoid overprotection. At the same time, the child should have good conversational skills and a healthy self-image.

SUMMARY

1. Deaf children with deaf parents have several advantages, in spite of the fact that their parents, on the average, have poorer education, a lower income, and poorer speech. The advantages were originally thought to be a result of earlier communication, but it seems that the parents' easier emotional acceptance of the child also plays a major role.

2. Many of the new ideas in early intervention are really old ideas that have been re-discovered.

3. There is still too little good evidence from scientific studies to show which are the most helpful and lasting components of early intervention.

4. Attention should be given to the emotional, informational, communication, and social needs of parents and children. The child should be considered a child first, with deafness and its management considered second.

5. Involvement of the entire family, including important relatives, is essential.

6. Services should be arranged so that responsibility, learning, and rewards include fathers and siblings.

7. Teachers of the deaf working in the home may be most aware of family needs, yet may have few counseling skills. These teachers need access to consultants.

8. A program is described that is based upon bicultural and bilingual principles. Important roles (including the directorship of the program) are assigned to deaf adults. There is flexibility in sign usage, rather than prescribing only one "correct" form.

Chapter 16

PRESCHOOL PROGRAMS

INTRODUCTION

In Chapter 15, *early* identification and *early* assistance for deaf children and their parents were stressed. There is no dispute about the importance of early intervention, but often it does not happen. We have already looked at some of the reasons for delay in diagnosis in Chapter 3. If the deafness is discovered fairly late (age two or three, for example), there may be insufficient time to do what is necessary before an early intervention program ends and preschool begins. Preschool programs can thus function either as extensions of early intervention efforts or as the first program a child and family encounter. Sometimes there is no organized program available between diagnosis and primary school age.

In North America, children enter regular or elementary school by age six. Many attend a kindergarten program at age five. The term "preschool" (sometimes referred to as "nursery school") would then refer to an educational group program prior to primary school entry (usually for children from ages three to five). Traditionally, children have been considered ready to separate from their parents and participate in group activities at about this age. Children younger than three, however, may be placed in day care programs because of their special needs or the needs of their working parents. (The program itself may differ for these younger children.)

Preschools usually last only two to four hours, whereas day care programs may keep children for an entire day. The preschool is usually more highly structured than the typical day care center. The latter will have rest or sleep time after lunch and more free play in the afternoon, when children tend to be too tired for a structured program. Sometimes both programs are combined: a child may be in a preschool program in the morning and remain in a day care program in the same or in another setting for the remainder of the day. The main differences between preschools and day care centers, then, concern the duration of the program and parental needs.

The terms used here, "preschools" and "day care," are primarily North American. Other terms may be used elsewhere.

This chapter examines some of the benefits of preschools for deaf children, the possibilities for integration of deaf children in regular preschools, some ideas for starting a preschool, and the role of deaf adults and parents (hearing and deaf) in school programs. We also consider how to provide your child with some of the same benefits of an organized preschool if one is not available in your community.

Because patterns of funding and legal requirements change frequently and differ from one area to another, we will not deal with these elements of school programs in detail.

WHAT PURPOSES DO PRESCHOOLS SERVE?

Children are usually enrolled in a preschool because their parents have certain needs or values: acceleration of their children's readiness for primary school, development of children's social skills, and need for time away from their children (because of work, other interests, or the burden of care).

For deaf children, there are other vital considerations: developing better communication, providing social contact with deaf (and hearing) children, and extending or beginning special services for child and parents (such as speech therapy, auditory training, and parent counseling). During a time of rapid development, deaf children urgently need to have their experiences "clothed with language," to use Lawrence Newman's phrase (personal communication, 1980). Thus, those who work with children in preschools (and many of the children's parents) do not consider these programs to be merely play groups or baby-sitting services.

Although some parents may be primarily concerned about the availability of a day care center so that they can work, for the staff the goals are very similar to those of preschools. Children are not just supervised; stimulating activities are organized in accordance with the children's ages.

Children may derive several benefits from a positive experience of separation from their parents, including: 1) development of skills to actively master their world, 2) consideration and attention to others, 3) cooperation with other children, 4) enjoyment of books, stories, and dramatic play, and 5) improvement in their muscular coordination. In this age range most children are not shy about using their bodies. They are open to all ways of communicating, including mime and sign language. Parents may be able to get a more objective idea than they previously had about how their child is learning and relating to others, and they can share their child's excitement in new experiences.

ARE TOTAL
COMMUNICATION PRESCHOOLS EFFECTIVE?

Probably the most complete follow-up study on the effectiveness of Total Communication preschools has been reported by Moores, Weiss, and Goodwin (1978; 1981, in press). The development of sixty children in seven different kinds of programs was followed for several years and many kinds of observations and assessments were made by people who did not know which program the child had attended.

A few of the results are of great importance. Although this was not an experimental study (as explained in Chapter 15), each educational program was examined in terms of the elements in it. It was found that, when added to amplified sound, each element (speechreading, fingerspelling, and signs) increased children's understanding. The Total Communication group, using a combination of amplification, speechreading, signs, and fingerspelling, was at the highest level of achievement in speech and academic readiness. Use of manual communication was not associated with less use of residual hearing or speechreading. Ratings done in the classrooms showed that the least two-way communication occurred in the auditory/oral program, and the most occurred in the program employing Total Communication.

Arnold and Tremblay (1979) observed the free play of six hearing and six deaf children in an integrated setting (described as Total Communication). Hearing children did not play as much with deaf children as with each other, and vice versa. The results of placement in integrated settings may therefore be mixed with regard to social interaction.

TYPES OF PRESCHOOLS

Preschools may be organized by the government (public), by a private agency or religious group, by a group of parents who each share certain responsibilities (a co-op), or by a service for handicapped children (clinic or child development center). Sometimes the preschools are combined with day care centers meeting the needs of working parents. The duration of the daily program is usually three to four hours because of the limited attention span of children of this age for a structured program.

THE DEAF CHILD IN ESTABLISHED PRESCHOOLS

In some communities it may be impractical to organize a specialized program because there are too few deaf preschool-age children. Several points should be considered. How much can a single deaf child profit from participating in a program for hearing children? The profit will probably not be much if there is no accommodation made for the child's deafness. Who will ensure that staff can communicate with the child? Will a teacher of the deaf come in periodically (an *itinerant teacher*) to advise the staff and improve their understanding? Where will related services be obtained (such as parent counseling)? Are opportunities provided for the hearing children to learn some signs? Could one or more of the staff learn signs?

The deaf child needs enough people (children and adults) with whom to communicate. This is difficult without the inclusion of other deaf children. Thus, the potential benefit for a deaf child attending a regular preschool for hearing children will depend upon preparing the staff so that both they and the hearing children can learn to communicate with signs. The presence of even one deaf adult signer has been found to increase deaf children's communication (Erting, 1978).

A NEW PROGRAM

If you are thinking of starting a preschool, you may be able to profit from the experience of others. For example, the International Association of Parents of the Deaf can advise you.

Adding a group of deaf children to an existing preschool or day care center has some advantages, because much of the initial work has already been done: facilities, board of directors, funding, and transportation arrangements already exist. On the other hand, there may be serious limitations in the attitudes of the staff or board toward deafness and deaf people. Often the staff need information and inservice training to help them understand the abilities and needs of children with hearing losses and how these qualities may differ from those of other "handicapped" children.

Enrolling the Children

Do not be overly optimistic. Although deaf children need opportunities, the number of parents who express interest in preschool programs or who claim that they will enroll their children is often inflated. Advertising for contacts with parents can be done in several ways: through organizations of deaf people, schools for the deaf, clinics, services for handicapped children, parent groups, and social and health agencies. The support of these groups can be important in obtaining funds, and it is worth spending time developing good relationships with them.

Obtaining Funds

Funds are sometimes provided by governments on a *per capita* basis—a set amount of money is paid for each child who attends. If one or two children drop out, income may decrease to the point at which the program cannot support itself. Parent fees are sometimes charged, but they usually are only a small part of the total.

Budgets may require some unusual items: interpreters for deaf persons attending parent and board meetings, staff training, and special equipment and acoustic treatment of the premises to control noise (on the advice of an audiologist). Conversion of physical facilities can be unexpectedly costly; thus, it is wise to obtain several good estimates before choosing a place in which to house your program.

Staff

There are varying local legal requirements for the ratio of staff to children in preschools, and for the training these people must have. In North America most preschool teachers have training in early childhood education and in child development, but they may not have a background in work with handicapped children. The staff in preschools for deaf children may have experience with deafness, but not in child development. The inclusion of both types of training is now becoming accepted as standard.

Preschool teachers and teachers of the deaf thus have different kinds of training, but both are important for preschool-age deaf children. At least one staff member should be a trained teacher of the deaf, and additional training and experience with preschoolers is desirable. Signing skills and knowledge about hearing aids, speech, and speechreading are fundamental for the other staff in a Total Communication program. A qualified deaf teacher or aide is strongly recommended as a role and language model (Erting, 1978).

Attitudes of staff toward deaf people, sign language, and spoken language should be assessed before hiring. Applicants should understand the goals and implications of Total Communication. Because children need pride in their developing communication skills, a sign-only or oral-only bias is limiting. Inexperienced hearing teachers are likely to give the deaf child an unintended message that only speech is important, while an overzealous sign language enthusiast may not provide adequate reinforcement for the development of speech, listening, and speechreading skills. A teacher who is flexible and knows his or her own limitations is usually preferable to one who has extensive experience but is rigid. Those who cannot communicate by means of signing and simultaneous communication will need formal training (courses), tutoring by deaf people, inservice training (lectures or seminars in your center), or all of these. Willingness to undertake these additional learning experiences is essential as a qualification for hiring.

Parent Involvement

Parents should be involved on the board of directors, on committees, in parent meetings with staff, and in the day-to-day program. Deaf parents (mothers *and* fathers) who have children in the program should be fully involved. This requires the provision of interpreters at meetings. Deaf parents are important models for both deaf and hearing preschoolers. It is an excellent idea to have them visit the class and help out just as the hearing parents do. A visit by you can indicate to your child that you value the program and take seriously what he or she is doing.

Parents enrolling their children need to receive a clear statement of the goals for their child and of the rules the parents and children are expected to follow (such as time of arrival and leaving, fees, required notice to withdraw from the program, and participation in meetings and in daily activities). A signed contract will help ensure that all parties are aware of mutual expectations.

Licensing Requirements

Licensing requirements may differ for different ages of children and different types of handicap. For example, fire regulations for deaf staff may be different. The assistance of a person from the licensing office is very helpful when starting a program.

Support and Consulting Services

When children become ill or have behavior problems, and when parents have special needs, additional help may be required. This may or may not be available locally through social or health agencies (private or governmental), or through clinic or hospital teams serving young deaf children. Consideration should be given to these needs during the early phases of organizing a preschool program.

Some way should be found to meet the needs of families for counseling and for communication skill development, either within the program or through a cooperative arrangement elsewhere. Schools for deaf children may be helpful by providing access to (or information about) books, courses, and audiovisual materials. Arrangements should also be made for periodic re-assessment of the children.

Board of Directors

Most preschools have their own board of directors who oversee the program. Involvement of both hearing and deaf parents is vital, and there should be at least one board member from the deaf community. Allowance for the costs of interpreters should be made. (If this is not done, most deaf people will not be able to participate effectively.) Persons trained in early childhood education and those who have deaf children of preschool age are valuable additions to a board of directors.

Transportation

Many programs survive or die based upon availability of transportation. Trips that seem short on the map can last longer than an hour or two when there are many side trips and stops. Because deaf children's homes may be widely scattered, there must be some way to get them to the preschool. Sometimes services for handicapped people will transport them. Parents cannot always bring their children, or if they can, they may not be able to retrieve them if the end of the preschool session is in the middle of the working day. Transportation responsibilities may be shared in a *car pool*. In most areas, volunteer drivers do not seem to be a satisfactory substitute because they cannot be depended upon. (This may nevertheless be feasible if there is a supervisor or coordinator of volunteers to accept responsibility.) Taxis have been a disaster in our experience (even if money is available to pay for them) because you never seem to get the same driver twice, the drivers don't usually understand deaf children, and they often can't deal with problems that arise. For all of these reasons, we advise a careful survey of transportation distances before a location for the preschool is chosen.

Other Considerations

Children considered for inclusion in a preschool program should be assessed for other problems that may affect the program, such as other disabilities or behavior problems. Deaf children with multiple disabilities may be acceptable in a home-based early intervention program, but on a group basis their needs may not be easily met without extra support services, staff training, and building alterations. It is our experience that, depending upon their special needs, these children should be considered for admission on an individual basis after the program is functioning smoothly. (We recognize a strong moral obligation to do whatever we can for special children and for their families, but not at the expense of other children.)

Preschoolers should be introduced to the program gradually, rather than all at once. This will allow staff to meet the parents, too.

Substitute staff should be available for staff illnesses, holidays, or professional development (conferences and courses). Insofar as possible, the substitute staff should be drawn from a small number of qualified personnel with whom the children may become familiar.

Deaf parents have a special interest in their children (hearing or deaf) attending a preschool organized for deaf children. An integrated setting can offer an excellent opportunity for the hearing relatives of a deaf child to gain more signing competence.

A TYPICAL DAY

The following description of a typical day in a preschool program refers to our own experience in Vancouver. Space restrictions prevent a full description, but it may be obtained upon request.

Following the usual greetings, the deaf children's hearing aids are checked and there is free play time with their deaf peers. Each child spends 10 minutes in an individual session with the teacher of the deaf, followed by art activity with scissors, glue, or paint. Various objects are matched during a math-readiness session. The children then engage in general play, such as building with large blocks or entertaining themselves in the dress-up corner. These activities are broken up with regular routines of toileting, clean-up, snacks, and quiet group time with the teacher. There may be a short neighborhood walk on which the children may look for signs of spring. Lunch with the hearing children is an opportunity to try out new signs with them, with each other, and with the staff, and perhaps to share secrets or to ask questions before leaving for home.

One of our teachers wrote: ". . . the child can try out different identities, activities, and behavior, take some risks, and see evidence of differing life-styles, personalities, and ways of doing things among children and adults. It is an exciting world with much to tell about, especially to mom and dad."

WHAT CAN YOU DO IF THERE ARE NO PRESCHOOLS?

The lack of preschools affects many parents who do not live in or near large population centers. Preschool can never take the place of home and family, but home, family, and community can largely replace preschool (T. Spradley, personal communication, 1980). What did parents do before there were any preschools? For socialization, they searched for other young deaf children and made sure the deaf children had a chance to play together. They arranged informal play groups and outings, and took turns babysitting or inviting their child's deaf friends for the weekend. For the development of communication skills, deaf adults or teenagers were sought. Use was also made of every available learning experience with hearing children and adults.

You may find one or all of these ideas useful, especially if you can think them through with other parents. Finding deaf people may be difficult at first, but persistence will pay off. The idea of contacting a deaf club or church in your area may make you nervous about your own communication skills, but once you have overcome your inhibitions, you will probably obtain many additional ideas and contacts that will help your child. The National Association of the Deaf and IAPD in the United States have a listing of clubs for deaf people and of parents who can serve as resources; similar services may be available in other countries.

If no services can be started because of lack of government interest, then parents must lobby to create support. Again, this is best done as a cooperative effort with the backing of deaf people and professional groups.

SUMMARY

1. Preschool or nursery school programs for deaf children are more than baby-sitting services. They provide an active learning experience in social, emotional, language, and intellectual areas. Usually they last from two to four hours and serve children between the ages of three and five.

2. Day care centers mostly serve children of working parents, tend to be somewhat less structured, and may keep the child for the entire day. Developmental goals are similar to those of preschools.

3. For deaf children, social contact with those who can communicate with them (other than family members) is essential. They need positive experiences of separation from their parents as well as access to the components of Total Communication.

4. Teachers of deaf children and preschool teachers often have different training backgrounds. They may need additional training if both are to function well in a preschool for children who are deaf.

5. It is difficult for a single deaf child to receive much benefit from a regular preschool unless there is considerable preparation of the staff and of the hearing children in the use of signs.

6. Adding a deaf program to an existing regular preschool has some advantages but also some disadvantages. The staff and board need to be educated, which requires openness and flexibility.

7. Starting a special program for deaf children that is organized from the beginning with their needs in mind may be the best available alternative. Necessary considerations that are discussed include: finding and enrolling the children, staffing, funding, parent involvement, inclusion of deaf people, the board of directors, transportation, consulting services, and children with multiple disabilities. It may be necessary for

parents to exert group pressure on government to
obtain needed help.

8. A combined preschool and day care center is
described. This arrangement has the advantage of
not depending entirely upon per capita funding
for a very small number of children.

9. When no preschool can be found or started, there
are still positive steps you can take: find other
deaf children for your child to play with, invite
deaf children to stay overnight or for a weekend,
use deaf adults or teenagers as baby-sitters, help
to provide a broad learning experience with
hearing children and adults, and write to your
national or regional associations of deaf people
and parents of deaf children for the names of
people with whom you can share experiences.

Chapter 17

LEARNING VACATIONS

Some parents commented that they really saw deaf people living their lives and being happy. It made them stop and think again and again . . . "I felt 'saturated' with deafness and very comfortable with it here, a feeling I hope won't leave. It made me realize how isolated I've been feeling at home. [p. 9] "We have been as close to our children's world as we ever can be. We want to make it our world." [Anonymous, 1974, p. 11]

INTRODUCTION

Several facts limit the possibilities of providing continuing services to all families with young deaf children: 1) there are so few deaf children that professional services and families tend to be widely separated from each other, 2) many of the needs of deaf children are difficult to meet through reading material and through occasional visits to professionals, 3) when the children are old enough to attend school the school system usually does not emphasize services for parents and siblings (which would be much later than is desirable), and 4) available services are likely to reach the mother alone and not other family members.

These are some of the reasons behind the learning vacation concept pioneered by Gallaudet College's Center for Continuing Education and the International Association of Parents of the Deaf in the summer of 1974 (Anonymous, 1974; Aldridge, 1980). These vacations have become increasingly popular and have now been held in several parts of the United States. In 1979, we independently established the first annual Total Communication learning vacation program in Canada, and another was independently organized at Donaldson's School for the Deaf in Edinburgh, Scotland. (Similar summer experiences had previously been available in the U.K. through the Breakthrough Trust.)

The Special School of the Future at Gallaudet College is willing to help with the establishment of new learning vacations (see address in back of this book.) Aldridge (1980) has also provided a thorough guide. Central to the success of all learning vacation programs are active parent participation, involvement of deaf people of various ages, and properly planned supervision for the children when they are away from their parents.

Gallaudet College and some other programs have offered learning vacations emphasizing: 1) the needs of multiply handicapped deaf children, 2) older deaf children (most programs have been for families of deaf infants and preschoolers), 3) attention to the needs of hearing siblings, and 4) child-rearing issues.

ADVANTAGES OF THE LEARNING VACATION PROGRAM

The arrangement of the learning vacation program over several days (usually five to ten days) enables families having little or no experience with deaf people to encounter them on a common level, perhaps for the first time. Because of the small size of the group (usually about 15 to 20 families), questions can be asked and feelings expressed in an informal, unhurried, supportive atmosphere. Many parents report that a learning vacation was their first opportunity to feel comfortable talking with professional people, such as audiologists and psychologists. For the professionals it also has advantages: they meet families without the usual pressure of time and they can understand how total families react more easily than is possible in their office practices. The result is that parents feel less alone with their feelings and professionals gain new insights.

CONTENTS OF THE PROGRAM

Sessions of the program led by professionals usually cover areas like the deaf community, causes of deafness, genetics, hearing and amplification, speech, child-rearing and discipline, and how to choose and evaluate an educational program.

Panel discussions have been very popular and helpful for parents. Panelists may include (in addition to hearing parents who usually have older deaf children) deaf adults who had deaf parents, deaf adults who had hearing parents, deaf parents with hearing children, and deaf parents with deaf children.

Sign language and simultaneous communication instruction (at different levels) are usually daily experiences for both parents and children. Deaf adults often serve as the instructors.

Additional elements of the program may include guest speakers, tours of schools in the area, and evaluations of children's hearing, hearing aids, and speech. The field trips and other leisure activities vary with the area and its offerings.

SUGGESTIONS FOR DEVELOPING A PROGRAM

The following program ideas are derived from our own experience, and may help to encourage total family attendance. Many other suggestions are contained in the new Gallaudet College handbook (Aldridge, 1980).

Funding may be obtained from several sources. Parent fees usually need to be at least partly subsidized, with arrangements made so that those families with very limited means may also attend. We suggest finding a service club or organization for the handicapped (not necessarily for deaf people) that will be interested in helping. Although most programs have been held at residential schools, ours has been in a summer camp setting some distance away from the city. (This has the advantage of less temptation to fragment the group process by going shopping, etc.) Some groups who have summer camps are willing to defray part of the costs. Government agencies may also be approached for funding.

Child care arrangements must be given high priority, or an otherwise excellent program can fail. Preferably, staff should be hired, rather than depending upon volunteers. Caring for hearing and deaf children of varying ages and making the program fun for them is hard work! Trained, experienced people should be involved in planning. Because of the social goals of the program, it is highly desirable to recruit deaf adolescents or young adults as child care staff.

Families with diverse backgrounds and varying degrees of experience are desirable, although those families whose sources of support are limited should be given priority. Seeing other parents coping well can be very reassuring.

It is advisable to have sign language instruction from deaf native signers. This ensures that parents will make efforts to communicate and to modify prejudices. (It is even better if the deaf instructors are familiar with manual codes and pidgin forms and have a balanced view of the different communication methods that may suit different deaf children.) Depending upon the orientation of those running the program, instruction and experience in simultaneous communication (such as manual code, pidgin forms, or cued speech) may also be included. On the other hand, if all parents have had instruction in a manual code, an emphasis upon a native sign language may be appropriate.

Vacant residential school buildings (including dormitories) have been used for some learning vacations. Some parents come from far away, using campers (recreational vehicles) or tents to reduce costs. Provision should be made for them to use their own sleeping accommodations, although they should be expected to eat with other participants in order to facilitate a favorable group process.

Invited speakers (from outside the area) should generally be carefully selected parents (hearing or deaf) with good skills in talking to groups, a sense of humor, and a broad, non-dogmatic view of the field.

Local speakers should not be chosen from only one center (school, hospital, or agency). It is better to promote cooperation among different groups rather than to maintain a "we can do everything" attitude. Using several representatives will require more planning and coordination. Speakers should be told what is expected of them and, if feasible, should have an opportunity to consult with the other speakers in the program.

Panel participants often have very interesting stories to tell. Videotaping is recommended if equipment is available, because the tapes may be used later as teaching and learning materials for those who did not attend.

It is particularly important to include deaf individuals who represent different ages of onset of deafness and varying levels of speech skills. When parents can laugh or cry at the story told by a non-speaking deaf adult, their idea that "success" and thinking are closely tied to speech are modified. *This is an essential point to consider.* One parent, after hearing a deaf panelist, spontaneously commented: "This is the first time I've felt proud to have a deaf child!"

It is important to schedule breaks and varied activities so that families do not become exhausted. The program is supposed to be a vacation, too!

Materials of interest to parents should be displayed: books, journals, and technical devices, such as TDDs (Telecommunication Devices for the Deaf), baby-cry alerts, and doorbells equipped with signal lights.

We suggest that special attention be given to the ways in which fathers, siblings, and relatives feel and function with the deaf child and the mother. This is a common area of concern for many families.

The learning vacation should foster parental awareness that they have needs *separate* from the field of deafness and from constant work with their deaf children. Parents themselves cannot and need not meet all their deaf children's needs.

Careful attention must be given to the question of including multiply handicapped deaf children in the learning vacation program. We are aware of their needs, which are often greater than those of ordinary deaf children, but these needs are less likely to be satisfied. It is also possible, however, that a learning vacation program of the type described will not meet multiply handicapped deaf children's needs unless special consideration and planning are undertaken. Their needs are so different that no general answer is possible. The concerns are: 1) much of the program may be unrelated to family needs if the child's additional disabilities are severe (if the child is so physically impaired or blind that sign language and/or speechreading will be impossible); 2) supervision of the child by child care staff may require special knowledge or procedures—these must be known before the child is accepted; and 3) the questions of the parents of multiply handicapped children may be by-passed in discussions because they represent concerns very different from those of all other families in the program. Simply knowing the medical labels of additional impairments is not helpful in making a decision. The program coordinator should ask what the parents expect to get out of the learning vacation and should get some idea of the child's developmental level before a fair decision on admission can be made. Some children with cerebral palsy, visual impairment, epilepsy, or mental retardation would definitely be appropriate. If there are enough multiply handicapped deaf children whose families wish to participate, organizing a special learning vacation with different content may be the best solution. Alternatively, a special day could be added to the regular program, or there could be some parallel programming.

Deaf culture should be included in the program. In many areas there are now deaf theater or mime groups, or solo deaf entertainers. Groups of deaf people should be familiar with these professionals. Culture should be discussed as a topic on the program: famous deaf people, what deaf groups have accomplished, and how deaf persons cope with everyday life situations. These activities are stimulating for young and older deaf children and their parents, and it is important to make good use of local deaf talent.

Hearing culture is equally significant, especially because it is a more difficult task for deaf children to acquire it. Ideas can be exchanged concerning how to help deaf children understand the way hearing people do things.

Finally, evaluation and feedback for the improvement of future programs should be collected from all participants before they leave.

CONCLUSIONS

If it is well planned, families will leave a learning vacation inspired by new knowledge, insights, attitudes, and friends. They will feel more confident in raising their deaf children as full members of their families and they will have acquired ideas about how to enrich their life experiences. Family ties may be strengthened. Parents will be better acquainted with sources of help. Above all, feelings about deafness and deaf people as human beings will be more realistic and positive.

It should also be noted that staff have needs, too. The warmth generated by an enthusiastic and appreciative group is a healthy incentive for them to continue their efforts and to improve their work.

SUMMARY

1. Learning vacations, if well organized and
    subsidized, offer an experience to many families
    (particularly those from rural areas) that cannot be
    provided as well in any other way.
2. Among the goals of such programs are: better
    communication of deaf children with their
    families; better parental understanding of
    language and other areas of child development;
    more positive attitudes toward deafness and deaf
    persons; having fun with deaf children while
    providing good learning experiences; and
    balancing family responsibilities.
3. Meeting deaf people on an equal basis is
    beneficial; involvement of deaf persons as sign
    language instructors, panelists, entertainers, and
    child care workers helps to provide models for
    the deaf child and broadens the family's
    understanding.
4. The inclusion of multiply handicapped deaf
    children in a program should be individualized
    because of their special needs.
5. Suggestions are given regarding funding, child
    care staff, and the contents of a new program.

Chapter 18

SCHOOLS
Ideology and Reality

The residential school provides the needed totality of experience, serves as the educational community, the social system, if you will, which is so necessary during the formative years for the development of self-concept and human relationships which carry over into adult life. [Garretson, 1977, p. 19]

. . . it's so institutionalized. I think that they've got to learn to live in a hearing world anyway, I mean, if they get too used to being with deaf people all the time, it will probably be harder to sort of fit in with the normal world . . . . [an English mother referring to a residential school, quoted in Gregory, 1976, p. 136]

INTRODUCTION

The issue of how schools can meet the needs of deaf children has continued to concern both parents and professionals. The remarks quoted above indicate that we should expect values and attitudes to be at least as important as facts in this field.

Education is also a controversial subject in regard to hearing children. Several major changes have been taking place over the past few years. People are skeptical that more, better, or different education can solve society's many problems. The new ideas that educators like to experiment with are being rejected in favor of a return to basic subjects and values. This movement is associated with the trend toward integrating handicapped children. Special classes and schools are often viewed in a negative light. The words now applied to special education have unpleasant associations: *segregated*, *restrictive*, *institutional*, *stereotyping*, and *stigmatizing*.

Education of deaf children is such a large and evolving subject that we need to restrict extended discussion to those topics that are not covered in materials easily available elsewhere. The references should provide sufficient additional sources of information. American parents should find the guide by Katz, Mathis, and Merrill (1978) helpful, and Evans (1977) has summarized the needs in Britain.

Some points to remember in reading this chapter are: 1) the focus is on severely and profoundly deaf children, not on those with lesser losses; 2) there is much individual variation even within this group; 3) because of the international audience to which this book is addressed and the continuing evolution of its implementation, the presentation of Public Law 94–142 in the United States will be brief; and 4) it should not be expected that a single "best" system for educating all deaf children can be described.

Many hard-of-hearing children receive no essential special services, although they constitute a much larger group than those who are deaf. Space limitations prevent us from dealing more with this important subject (see Davis, 1977). (The contents of this book are most relevant to profoundly prelingually deaf children and are less applicable to those children in which the severity of deafness decreases and age of onset of hearing impairment increases.)

Our presentation of education for deaf children is best considered as a stimulus to thinking rather than as a final and adequate summary of a large and changing field.

USE OF TERMS

Educators and administrators, like other professionals, tend to use a lot of *jargon*, or technical language, sometimes in confusing ways. When you are in doubt about the meaning of a word or phrase, we suggest that you request clarification.

Perhaps the two most important words receiving recent attention are *integration* and *mainstreaming*. Sometimes the words are used interchangeably, sometimes distinctions are made between them, but essentially they refer to activities in which deaf children join hearing children. Often main-streaming is used to mean full integration. The word comes from the concept of different "streams" of education: the mainstreamed deaf child would thus be in the main, or normal majority stream. (Another expression is "decentral-ization," referring to the establishing of local or regional programs instead of, or in addition to, a centralized facility.)

CONFUSION OF DEAFNESS WITH OTHER DISABILITIES

Unfortunately the field of education is not exempt from the general tendency to lump deafness with other disabilities or "handicaps." If a plan or approach is good for one or more kinds of disabled children, then it is likely to be viewed as equally good for all. People who are not familiar with deafness may have little or no appreciation of the fact that the effects of deafness are unlike those of other disabilities.

WHAT DO PARENTS WANT MOST?

Parents want to feel confident that their child is happy, is in the right school, and is making satisfactory academic and social progress. Educational theories may seem far removed from daily life, but parents need some awareness of how theories lead to actual changes in programs.

The parents of hearing children are also concerned about education, but they are more likely to have options. The very small number of deaf children in most communities (one or two per 1,000 children) limits choices and program flexibility and can result in serious conflicts between parents and educators.

WHAT ARE THE AIMS AND TASKS OF EDUCATION?

Children's skills in thinking and self-reflection develop rapidly during the school years. They are expected to sit still, pay attention, be motivated, obey rules, cooperate with their peers, delay satisfactions, and in general do what others want them to do. However, more is involved than learning to conform and obey: this is also a time of creativity and of wonder about the world, if these feelings are not stifled. "Education aims toward a healthy self-concept for each child—in short, development of the whole person" (Garretson, 1977, p. 20).

Hockenhull has emphasized that the challenge to teachers of the deaf is to:

> . . . develop in our children those inner resources and attitudes that will help them to live rich, satisfying lives . . . It is not enough that they should merely exist . . . The first quality that we must give to deaf children is a sense of wonder; that is, the ability to perceive and to relish the things around him. . . . [Hockenhull, 1979, p. 99]

Garretson (1977) estimated that about 92% of a child's time is spent out of the classroom. This is the non-school aspect of learning, which he terms the "unwritten curriculum." More time is spent watching television, sleeping, and eating than in class, but despite this fact, the school is an important influence. It is through the "unwritten curriculum" that much learning takes place, but the deaf child (especially of hearing parents) may be deprived of broad learning opportunity. How can the community be a real influence for the deaf child? According to Garretson, it may be "a physical presence but a mental blankness," with the child "a silent member of the crowd, present and yet absent, a second-class participant with latent leadership abilities undeveloped and dormant without much of a chance to contribute" (p. 20).

HOW DO DEAF CHILDREN COMPARE WITH HEARING CHILDREN IN ACHIEVEMENT?

As a group, deaf children are substantially behind hearing children in school achievement, even if they are of equivalent intelligence. Conrad (1979) gave tests to almost every graduate of classes for deaf children in England and Wales (well over 500 children). Some of his findings were mentioned briefly in Chapter 10, but are worth reporting in more detail here. On a standardized test of reading comprehension, only five deaf children reached the average level of reading for hearing children (and two of these children had deaf parents). More than 70% of profoundly deaf graduates had speech that was rated by their own oral head teachers as very difficult or impossible to understand; this was confirmed by independent tests. Their speechreading ability was at about the same level as inexperienced hearing volunteers of the same age. (Try turning off the sound on your television set and seeing how much you can understand.)

There were two factors that influenced high scores on these tests: degree of hearing loss and IQ. The best way to be "an oral success," Conrad pointed out, is to be very bright and not very deaf. Other surveys from the United States generally confirm these findings (Jensema et. al., 1978; Moores, 1978b).

One major difficulty in determining achievement in deaf children has been the use of inappropriate tests that are designed for hearing children and that require a good knowledge of written English. Even when appropriate tests are used, however, performance tends to be poor, especially in reading. There has been much speculation about the reasons for this, but the reading process is still not well understood, even in hearing children. The subject has been reviewed by Brooks (1978) and by Gallaudet College (1979).

The average reading ability of deaf secondary school graduates is at about the level of grades three to five, meaning that many deaf adolescents and adults are functionally illiterate and cannot read for pleasure. Although some improvement can be obtained by intensive training later, little if any advance usually occurs during the later school years. (This is a compelling reason to provide better programs at earlier ages.) It does seem that lack of constant and natural two-way use of the surrounding spoken language is one factor. Many believe that the early introduction of signing in order to acquire a first language will improve achievement in communication, but it is too early to make sweeping claims. More evidence should be available soon.

One fact is often overlooked: *many deaf people know much more than is indicated by their performance on tests.* Caution is certainly needed before labeling a deaf child as "mentally retarded," as a "slow learner," or as "low verbal."

SCHOOLS AND CULTURE

If by "culture" we mean the sum total of the rules, values, and expectations by which we make sense of our particular environment, then schools have their own culture. To some degree each school has an individual culture (most obvious with some of the well-known and prestigious private schools), and to a smaller degree each class or grade will differ. Homes and schools share many of the common values of the larger culture of society, but not all of them. Differences between home and school often cause misunderstandings between parents and educators, and the children are caught in the middle.

Suppose that your teenager refuses to wear certain clothes to school that you feel should be acceptable. If you demand an explanation, you are likely to be told that you don't understand or that "no one would be caught dead in something like that!" Although you may never have used the term, you have met a very clear example of *cultural* differences.

In a painstaking study of 12 English secondary schools, Rutter and his colleagues (1979; summarized in Rutter, 1980) were able to demonstrate that the schools had a marked effect on their students, part of which was cultural. The outcome in behavior and attainment was better for those schools that, as a social system, encouraged students to accept responsibility, that provided incentives, and that were convinced that their students could do well. These findings are probably equally important for deaf children, who may be unintentionally excluded from important and beneficial influences in some hearing schools (Farrugia and Austin, 1980).

You may consider the culture of your child's school to be good or bad, but probably you are only aware of a few superficial aspects of it from your adult point of view. If your child is "left out" and not a part of the school culture, life may be very difficult. Peer group rules and expectations are at least as powerful as those set by teachers and parents, especially in adolescence (Farrugia and Austin, 1980).

John, profoundly deaf, attended a residential school during the primary grades. His parents missed him and, encouraged by several professionals, they decided to mainstream him in the local high school with some itinerant help in spite of his poor speech. Within a few months he was in social difficulties. He attended a dance and was left out; his approaches to hearing girls were rebuffed. He became increasingly lonely, frustrated and depressed. Return to the residential school proved to be the only option in this instance.

Until relatively recently, most deaf children attended a special school, either day or residential, where they could be a fully functioning part of their school and class culture. Many deaf adults can tell you how important residential school was to them *socially*, whether the school was good academically or not. They recount endless anecdotes, both amusing and sad. They were a *part* of these experiences that contributed to their personality and sense of group identity. Those involved in designing programs or in arranging placements should take into consideration whether the deaf child in question can be a part of the school culture.

WHAT DO DEAF CHILDREN NEED?

Deaf children have the same needs as hearing children, but these may sometimes be better satisfied in special ways.

At the same time that hearing children are learning academic subjects with substantial content, deaf children are typically struggling to achieve a working knowledge of

English. Their teachers spend much of their time teaching the spoken and written language and correcting errors, most of which are self-correcting for hearing children. This is one reason that deaf students on the average are far behind their hearing peers. The lag is greatest in subjects requiring knowledge of the spoken language (such as English or social studies), less severe in mathematics, and least problematic in expressive subjects like art and physical education. Yet the need to acquire information about the world around them is no less for deaf children.

Deaf children also need to be able to communicate with their teachers. Suppose your hearing child came home and reported to you: "My teacher can't understand English." There would probably be quick action from outraged parents, but this situation has been a *normal* one for deaf children, and hardly anyone seems outraged! Recently a judge in Chicago ruled that it is discriminatory for a white teacher not to understand and speak Black English to a class of black children. Teachers with children who use a different language or dialect may have to learn that form in order to teach Standard English. (Black English is a dialect that has only recently been considered worth studying. Linguists discovered that it is a full dialect, not a degenerate form of Standard English.) What would happen if a similar recognition were given to sign languages and sign codes? Teachers of deaf children would actually be able to communicate with them without difficulty! The obstacle here is that, unlike black children whose parents share their dialect, most deaf children have hearing parents, who are unlikely to champion a language (or mode) in which they are not fluent and about which they know little.

It is more difficult for hearing teachers to serve as good models for deaf children if they can't communicate freely and if they don't understand how the deaf child sees the world. Deaf teachers are usually the most popular with deaf children; we consider this to be natural and unavoidable.

Parents also need to improve their communication skills and understanding of deafness during their children's school years. School systems should provide for this (Schein, 1977), but many do not yet do so.

THE CONCEPT OF INTEGRATION

Background

There are at least three sources of the enthusiasm surrounding integration: 1) an understandable parental wish to have the child live at home (or closer to home), rather than have him or her attend a residential school; 2) a strong movement to include handicapped children (originally children who were mildly mentally retarded) in mainstream education; and 3) well-intentioned, but perhaps misguided, efforts by legislators to reduce the costs of centralized schools by placing the responsibility for special education on local authorities.

Brill, Merrill, and Frisina (1973) have emphasized the need for large enough groups of deaf children to make local specialized programs feasible. These researchers estimate that a minimum of 40 children is needed for an elementary program and 150 children for a secondary program. There should be a maximum class size of six for preschool and primary grades, eight for elementary, and ten for secondary schools.

Justification for these figures is based on the need for personnel and services (trained teachers, supervisors, and support specialists); parent, personal, and vocational counseling; a variety of program possibilities; and a maximum travel time to and from the school of 45 minutes each way for elementary students and 60 minutes each way for secondary students.

A community would need to have approximately 40,000 children to supply this minimum number of elementary students and 150,000 children to supply enough secondary pupils. This is a substantial population base, and is one reason why it was necessary to establish residential schools in the first place.

Different Kinds of Integration

In his survey of mainstreaming programs for prelingually deaf children in the United States, Brill (1978) identified four main patterns: 1) deaf children are based in *regular* classes with teachers not trained in deafness, and they receive limited help from a teacher of the deaf (itinerant teacher) one or more days a week; 2) although they are based in a *regular* class, part of the children's time is spent in a resource room with a teacher of the deaf (usually daily); 3) the base class is a *special* class, but for one or more academic subjects they join hearing children; and 4) the integration is only in non-academic classes (such as art and physical education). A variation of integration is team teaching in a regular class with one of two teachers being a teacher of the deaf (Kopchick, 1977). Various arrangements with interpreters may also be made, although this is not generally as satisfactory as having a teacher who signs.

Some residential schools partially integrate their students in neighborhood schools; they may also have hearing children come to their school part of the time.

Public Law 94–142 in the United States

In 1975 the Education for All Handicapped Children Act was passed, guaranteeing a free, appropriate, and individualized education for each handicapped child from age three through age 18 (extended to age 21 in 1980). State and local educational agencies receive federal money based upon a count of handicapped children in their area (this encourages locating children who are not being served). The rights granted parents are extensive: to be informed of all decisions affecting identification, evaluation, placement, and programming; to participate in decision-making; to accept or reject findings and decisions; and to challenge these actions through "due process" legal procedures. There are additional rights to confidentiality of records and non-discriminatory testing (related to race, culture, language, or communication method).

The most controversial provision, especially for children who are deaf, is the right to education in the "least restrictive environment" (IAPD, 1979).

A central part of the plan is the Individualized Education Program, or IEP. This is a written statement, prepared at least annually, which includes the child's present level of performance, annual goals and short-term objectives to meet these goals, specific services to be provided (including extent of integration), and the way in which progress towards objectives will be determined. The IEP must be prepared jointly by qualified staff and the parents, with the student participating if this is appropriate. Thus, the plan cannot be "sprung" on the parents by surprise, and records can be examined before the conference. Parents have the right to an interpreter, if necessary, at public expense. Schools are held responsible for cooperation in good faith, but not for guaranteeing success. (The IEP document is not a legal contract.)

Gallaudet College has published an excellent parent guide on Public Law 94–142 (Rosen, 1979).

The implications of the "least restrictive environment" are controversial. Handicapped children are required to attend programs for non-handicapped children *if this is judged to be beneficial for the child*. This immediately raises the old controversy over the "deaf world," the "hearing world," segregation, integration, and deaf culture. It seems that some parents, educators, and administrators have misunderstood the law to mean that mainstream education is *necessarily* the "least restrictive environment," when, for many deaf children, it may be the *most* restrictive (IAPD, 1979; Vernon, 1975). Although a few deaf children can fully compete with hearing children in a regular class, and can integrate socially, this is unusual and is not something one can expect.

It should be understood that it is the burden of the educator to prove that a residential or special day program is superior to an integrated setting. Legal challenges to Public Law 94–142 as it applies to deaf children are under way. An official resolution of the Council for Exceptional

Children (North America) in 1980 emphasized that alternatives *must* be maintained and that the "least restrictive environment" refers to more than the physical or geographical location of an educational program.

What are Some of the Problems
with Integration, or Mainstreaming?

An excellent review by Nordén and Ang (1980) has been published by the National Swedish Board of Education. Their conclusion is that:

> The total picture of studies focusing on the effects of school placement on hearing-impaired pupils is that we as yet have grossly incomplete knowledge of the pupils' situation. [p. 30]

Brill (1978) reported the comments of teachers and administrators in various kinds of integrated programs in the United States. First we look at a few of their negative comments:

> The deaf students get along with the hearing students on a casual level. They are rarely ever accepted as an integral part of the group in its social life. [p. 34]

> It was observed that a child in a hearing class with an interpreter was really in the second most restrictive environment. The most restrictive environment is the deaf child in a class without an interpreter. With an interpreter, communication is almost exclusively from the teacher to the pupil . . . the interpreter does not have time to explain what is being said. There is very little reverse interpreting from pupil to teacher. There is even less communication between pupil and pupil if interpreting is required. [p. 88]

> [In another program,] . . . the administrator said he had made an analysis of the number of times a regular teacher had communicated with the hearing impaired child in the class, and that it was only three times over a very long period. He thought this was rather typical; that in many instances the hearing impaired child was not really involved in what was going on in the class. [p. 111]

Reduction in class size to compensate for the extra time a teacher must spend with a mainstreamed deaf child has been considered essential, but seems uncommon.

There were also positive comments about integration: better opportunities to make friends in the home neighborhood, better models of behavior, and more challenging academic teaching for bright deaf children.

Greenberg and Doolittle (1977) have expressed the following concerns about mainstreaming:

1. Local regular class and special education teachers are not adequately trained to have deaf children in their classes.
2. Living at home may mean poor communication with the family, loneliness, and social isolation. Most rapid, easy communication between hearing people is not understood by deaf children.
3. If interpreters are provided, there still may be problems. There may not be enough interpreters, or they may have to function also as tutors, teaching concepts that are taken for granted by hearing children while trying to interpret new classroom material. Much social communication cannot be interpreted at all.
4. Where will the specialized supervisors and support staff come from? For example, psychologists need special training to test a child who is deaf.
5. If only the "problem children" remain in a centralized school, funding may go to the brightest and best-adjusted children in integrated settings, leaving the centralized schools with shrunken budgets to meet their students' needs. It may be more difficult to justify specialized support staff when the number of children in the schools decreases.
6. Evaluation of children's progress, once they are dispersed, may be difficult. How will overall problems with the plan be identified and remedied?
7. What kind of help can be offered to families when only a small number of children are in a district?
8. Will hearing classmates get sufficient preparation, so that real acceptance of deaf children can become a reality?
9. Most of the people designing and implementing local programs have little, if any, awareness of deafness and of deaf people, of deaf culture, and of the importance of deaf teachers.

It seems clear that narrow interpretations by administrators and legislators of what deaf children need may pose serious risks to their development (Convention of American Instructors of the Deaf, 1980; Vernon, 1975).

Who Are the Deaf Children in Mainstream Programs?

According to Karchmer and Trybus's survey of the United States (1977), students in integrated programs tend to have less severe hearing losses and more intelligible speech, and they come from families with higher incomes and better education. For example, two-thirds of those in residential schools were profoundly deaf, but this was true of only 18% of those in integrated settings. Of all profoundly deaf children, only 8% were in integrated classes. (Most postlingually deafened children were mainstreamed.) Of children with deaf parents, most attended residential schools by preference.

Reich, Hambleton, and Houldin (1977) tested 195 hearing-impaired children in integrated settings in the Toronto area, most of whom were found to be hard-of-hearing. The few apparently successful *deaf* children had good speech and speechreading, but still required intensive, specialized support. Integration seemed to have some academic benefits, but the researchers were concerned about personal and social difficulties. Similar findings for schools in the United States were reported by Karchmer, Milone, and Wolk (1979). However, integrated children had individual differences before the programs began; therefore, success cannot be attributed to the mainstreaming itself (Moores et al., 1981, in press).

What are the Needs of a Local Program?

The needs outlined by Brill et al. (1973) include acoustically treated rooms, hearing aid maintenance, trained supervisors, and an experienced support staff (audiologists, speech therapists, psychologists). The specific needs will vary depending upon whether the local program consists of special classes, mainstreaming, or both. Nix (1977) has developed a Mainstream Placement Question/Check List of items to consider before a deaf child is mainstreamed. This list includes:

average or better learning rate; ability to comprehend spoken directions and follow large group discussions; willingness to ask questions for clarification; language, social, and emotional development; reading level comparable to that of hearing children; academic skills within one grade level of others in the class; resilient personality; at least average self-control; ability to relate well to hearing adults and peers; and speech intelligible enough to be understood by the teacher and peers. Very few deaf children fullfill these requirements.

OTHER EDUCATIONAL NEEDS

Because many deaf children are still deprived of much common knowledge, they have an even greater need for what is sometimes termed "family life education," which includes sex education (Caley and Gibson, 1978; Fitz-Gerald and Fitz-Gerald, 1976). Deaf children's opportunities to learn from their hearing parents and siblings and from conversations and television may be severely curtailed. They may "overhear" little, and therefore cannot ask obvious questions, and their experimentation with the opposite sex may also be limited. They need to learn about the feelings of others and about responsibility just as much as about the physical "facts of life."

Sex education is now being taught in a few centralized schools (North Carolina Schools for the Deaf, 1979), but better ways need to be found to include this experience in other types of educational settings. The program in our Provincial school (Jericho Hill School for the Deaf) illustrates one plan. Small co-educational groups of about ten boys and girls meet with a male and a female teacher. If the topic makes the children uncomfortable, the boys and girls may separate. Subjects that are less emotionally loaded are considered first (different life-styles, leaving home). No knowledge concerning sexuality can be taken for granted. Instructors need to be comfortable with the subject matter and with very direct personal questions. An appreciation of different points of view and the reasons behind them is encouraged.

Another essential area of knowledge is the world of work: how to open a bank account, pay taxes, buy a car, fill out a job application, and tolerate boring work while waiting for a more stimulating position. These skills are probably at least as important as the usual academic subjects. Special attention must be given to those experiences that have been missed because of lack of incidental learning. The best example we have seen of a teaching guide to the rules of life (from buying a used car and attending a funeral to politely declining a written invitation) was produced by the Victorian School for Deaf Children in Melbourne, Australia (Murkin and Womersley, 1978). It is an attempt to explain what you can expect (and what is expected of you) as a member of society. Similar guides should be produced elsewhere that take national differences into consideration.

Many deaf teenagers wish to further their education after graduation. Until recently, university attendance was rare because there was no organized support system, but this is now changing. Interpreters and note-takers are being made available within college and university settings in several countries. The United States is favored with the best facilities in the English-speaking world. Among them are Gallaudet College, the world's only liberal-arts college for deaf people, which accepts many foreign students, and which is supported by direct Congressional funding; the National Technical Institute for the Deaf; and the new Southwest College for the Deaf in Texas. There are also various regional centers. Parents of deaf children should know about Gallaudet College as a world center of deaf learning (see Figure 10). *Gallaudet Today* is the best single source of information.

A free guide to North American college and career programs for deaf students is available (Rawlings, Biser, and Trybus, 1978). Information for other countries may be obtained through national organizations.

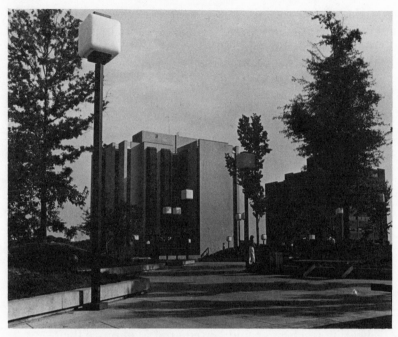

Figure 10. Gallaudet College campus: College plaza with dormitories. [Courtesy of Charles Shoup and Gallaudet College.]

SOME THOUGHTS ON AN "IDEAL" BILINGUAL PROGRAM

Moores (1978a) has described a gap between educational research and practice. Few educational practices have been well evaluated prior to their implementation. In this section we present some ideas about bilingual programs based upon other concepts and facts outlined in this book. We don't claim that these practices will necessarily solve all problems.

The real issue, according to Stokoe, is:

> . . . not oralism *vs.* manualism, as much time has been wasted arguing; instead the issue is whether the true bilingual situation of the deaf—Sign *and* English—is to be recognized. The question to be faced by all who have a hand in shaping the life circumstances of the deaf is this: will the deaf person reach maximum competence in English better if forced into apparent monolingual use of English or if the need for bilingual development is acknowledged and satisfied? [Stokoe, 1980, p. 147]

Kannapell (1974) has discussed bilingualism and its relationship to schooling. ASL has had almost no official place in schools for deaf children: "Neglect of the language of deaf persons is accompanied by a neglect of their history and culture" (p. 14). In order to establish an "ideal" day or residential school program, we would suggest consideration of the following ideas set out by Kannapell for those children who have had the benefits of early intervention and pre-school programs:

1. *Respect for native sign language.* Students should use (or learn to use) and develop their skills through interaction with deaf teachers and other staff as well as with peers. Art forms, theater, poetry, mime, and story-telling are highly valued as important expressive abilities. The pride of deaf children in their language is a fundamental part of the school's atmosphere. This requires a significant proportion of qualified deaf staff in the program and the support of hearing teachers. Although they themselves may never acquire expressive fluency in the native sign language, hearing teachers should be required to improve their signing skills.

2. *Deaf studies program.* Heroes, history, the nature of deafness, and how deaf people cope with life should be presented (Schein, 1977).

3. *English as a second language.* Teaching of English is a very important part of the curriculum, not through repetitive remedial drill but through modern concepts of second language learning. For this to succeed, the hearing teachers need an understanding of the structure of sign language (Goldberg and Bordman, 1975).

4. *Teaching and development of ASL and English.* The study of ASL and English should be coordinated, but the languages probably should be presented separately, at least part of the time.

5. *Use of hearing aids, auditory stimulation techniques, speech articulation improvement, and speechreading.* These methods are a part of the curriculum, but are employed in a manner that doesn't overemphasize what the student cannot do. If no reasonable progress is made, one or more of these approaches is abandoned as non-productive.

6. *Manually coded sign systems.* Manual codes are employed flexibly when needed to convey the properties of English.
7. *Integration.* Sharing of activities with hearing children is encouraged, but only under conditions likely to benefit the student. The school itself should be such an exciting place that some hearing students would want to integrate *there.*
8. *Family involvement.* Family communication is assessed and improved where necessary.

CONCLUSIONS

We have tried to describe the present situation in schools for deaf children, as well as possibilities for the future. It is difficult for us to see how mere placement of deaf children in a local school setting can be expected to accomplish anything other than temporarily hiding the child's increasing social, academic, and linguistic impoverishment. Although a few profoundly or severely deaf children with exceptional skills may succeed, present evidence suggests that this is possible only for a small minority. Thus, although the concept of integration has some positive aspects, there are real dangers unless very careful planning is undertaken.

Acceptance of deafness as a condition with cultural and social effects (many of which are positive) leads to an educational design (such as Kannapell's) different from the approach that emphasizes defect. However, we still do not know the benefits of putting into practice a program that deals with the social-cultural effects of deafness; it has yet to be done. In light of the rapid advances made recently by many children, it is our belief that such social-cultural effects should be seriously considered, and that many of the school achievement problems described in this chapter might be overcome as a result.

Educators and parents have a mutual responsibility to work toward equalized opportunities for deaf children in both the written and "unwritten" curriculum and to ensure that appropriate options are not lost. There are better reasons for maintaining options than merely to satisfy squabbling parents, professionals, and deaf persons. Deaf children and their families have different needs and skills. Much more can and must be done to evaluate and to improve special schools (residential and day), special classes in ordinary schools, and integrated settings before any one option is either eliminated or made mandatory. We caution that this assessment must be done without making deaf children feel that their self-worth depends upon losing their deafness. Such an attitude is more difficult to avoid in integrated settings.

SUMMARY

1. Recent changes in the education of handicapped children are affecting deaf children, although this may be unfortunate in many ways. These changes include an emphasis on integration or mainstreaming, which reduces the importance of the centralized special school.
2. Education is more than formal schooling. Thought must also be given to how deaf children can make the most productive and enjoyable use of the "unwritten curriculum" outside of class.
3. An important aim of education is a healthy self-concept, which is developed by using the child's skills and abilities to increase awareness of the wonder and workings of the world.
4. The school achievement of deaf children (reading, speech intelligibility, and speechreading), on the average, is quite disappointing. This is not the same, of course, as measuring success in life.
5. Many deaf people know more than the usual tests can show.
6. Schools have their own set of rules and attitudes—their culture. It is important for deaf children to feel a part of the school culture, which is difficult if they can't understand most of what is happening.
7. Deaf children need good communication with their teachers; often this is not achieved.
8. Integration is not new, but has been practiced in one form or another for many years. It often fails to fulfill expectations. Several kinds of integration are described. All require expensive and extensive support services. A major problem is that most school systems have no place for deaf teachers.
9. Public Law 94–142 is described briefly as the most extensive attempt to provide free education for handicapped children. There are still many problems in its application to deaf children.

10. Social isolation in the midst of "integration" is common.

11. Children who are integrated have more hearing, show higher IQs, are better educated, come from higher income families, and have more intelligible speech. It is likely that only relatively few deaf children can be mainstreamed, although contact with hearing children can be beneficial.

12. An "ideal" school approach is described that emphasizes deaf culture, language, and pride equally with English and academic subjects, but the program has yet to be adequately tried.

Chapter 19

PARENTS AND PROFESSIONALS AS PARTNERS

No one is more concerned about a deaf child than the parents. But in most cases parents have no idea how to go about effectively getting the services their child needs. And often there are unresolved feelings of guilt and hostility that influence the way parents proceed. Who better to vent these feelings on than a teacher, administrator, or doctor who seems to show no concern or who is not providing services at—in a parent's view—a reasonable level of quality? It is difficult to negotiate effectively in this type of circumstances. [T. Spradley, personal communication, 1980]

INTRODUCTION

Parents and those working with deaf children often share common goals and have common views of how to reach those goals. In this sense there is a natural partnership, one that can be very satisfactory—but partners do not always agree. The measure of a true partnership lies not in total agreement, but in how the relationship endures and grows in spite of differences.

Much has been written about how professionals should treat parents and why parents act the way they do. Little information is available to parents to help them understand professionals and to assist them in developing constructive ways to bring about the changes that seem necessary. In this chapter we examine the parent-professional relationship. No sweeping generalizations are intended: we see no villains or conspiracies. Both parents and professionals can be reasonable and can have good intentions, but they can still disagree.

263

They can both be overly emotional, short-sighted, impulsive, rigid, defensive and unreasonable, too.

    We will focus mostly on the ways in which parents can solve problems, but this is not meant to indicate that most problems are the fault of professionals.

GENERAL PROCEDURES ADVISABLE FOR PARENTS

Before considering specific types of problem-solving, parents should generally do the followings things: 1) acknowledge positive things and helpful people; 2) show a willingness to listen to other points of view; 3) request clarification of disputed decisions or policies, in writing if necessary; 4) keep good records of important phone calls and conferences, and follow them up with a letter of understanding; 5) discuss negative feelings with others *before* acting on them; and 6) act jointly with parent organizations when problems are wide-reaching and important.

THE SOURCES OF PROBLEMS

Introduction

No one really expects complex human problems to yield to simple approaches. Problem-solving techniques must be suited to a diagnosis of the disordered relationships between parents and professionals. Here we present one way of looking at the sources of difficulty and suggest the kinds of approaches that might help solve conflicts.

Differing Priorities

Parents are interested in their own child; educators and administrators are interested in many children. *Conflict*: The parent wants a teacher re-assigned when the present distribution of students and teachers seems to be the best compromise. *Possible solutions*: Make the best case you can, including a description of how the situation is affecting your child's attitude toward school; find out who sets priorities; if necessary, go to higher authorities or get an independent professional opinion.

Knowledge of Deafness and Deaf People

You may feel that your personal experience is worth 20 years of training, but don't expect all professionals to agree; they may have out-of-date knowledge but find it impossible to admit this. *Conflict*: You believe it is important to have deaf adults as teachers or as other staff in the school and the principal can't understand why you are so radical. *Possible solutions*: Inquire politely about the person's background in the area of deafness concerned, or about who is making the decisions; indicate that the issue is controversial, and that new methods are rapidly advancing; offer information from your own investigations and be very clear on your reasons for wanting deaf staff or other changes.

Gaps in Information About Child's Current Situation

People create meaning from the information available, but this information is always limited. *Conflict*: A school principal acts on the assumption that what a teacher reports is correct or that no further information is necessary; a parent, as in the example above, assumes that the teacher is wrong because the child's reported behavior is not evident at home; a physician accepts the child's office behavior as an adequate indication of what happens in outside settings. *Possible solutions*: Consider the possibility that you may not have adequate information (no matter how sure you are), and then get more information.

Beliefs, Feelings, Assumptions, and Fears about Education

Beliefs, feelings, assumptions, and fears may underline differing interpretations of "facts." *Conflicts*: Controversies over methods of communication, "deaf and hearing worlds," expectations for deaf children. *Possible solutions*: there are no simple solutions. Persuasion, re-education, use of other experts, and pressure to change policies if negotiation is impossible are some possible actions.

Style and Personality

People often react solely on the basis of the style with which others approach them. *Conflict*: A parent sensitive to the apparently condescending approach of a professional takes offense and reacts impulsively and abrasively, making later compromise or change difficult or impossible. *Possible solutions*: Try not to make people express extreme opinions too quickly, leave room for compromise; write down and discuss actions first; if necessary, admit that the initial meeting was unfortunate and try to start over.

Past Experiences

Having good (or bad) experiences with deaf children, parents, deaf people, or professionals may bias later reactions. *Conflict*: The parent reacts to a new person by thinking: "he reminds me so much of . . ." or "I know her type!" *Possible solutions*: Try to become aware of what it is that you don't like about a person and consider whether that person's similarities to a previous acquaintance are really that significant.

Pressures from Elsewhere

Decisions or policies may not be the ultimate responsibility of the person with whom you are disagreeing. *Conflict*: Political and financial pressures may be put on school boards; personal problems of parents that are not revealed, such as conflicts with spouse or relatives, may be affecting their attitudes. *Possible solutions*: Find out where the outside pressures are coming from and go to the source to relieve them.

Not Understanding the System

If you don't know how school hierarchies, medical teams, or other organizations work, you can easily misinterpret what happens or become known as a trouble-maker. *Conflict*: You complain to a clinic director without first talking with the professionals concerned. *Possible solutions*: Always try to resolve issues directly; talk with others to find out how things work; but don't let a complicated bureaucratic run-around keep you from getting satisfaction.

THINGS TO AVOID IN RELATIONS WITH PROFESSIONALS

The following useful points concerning relations with professionals are modified from a list compiled by Thomas Spradley (personal communication, 1980):

1. Don't make threats.
2. Offer solutions that leave room for compromise: "Here is what we think should be done to help Johnny succeed. If there is something here that you can't live with, we are open to your suggestions."
3. When you feel anger and hostility, recognize that at least some of it has nothing to do with the individual with whom you are dealing.
4. Perspective comes from talking with other parents. If you think you are the only person with a particular problem it will be easy for a professional to make you think you are unreasonable.
5. Don't talk about other children, other parents, or other teachers; don't allow the professional with whom you are dealing to make comparisons either.
6. Visit your child's class regularly. When you show interest and concern for your child *and* for the school and teacher, the facility and staff will reflect your interest and concern.
7. Remember that a problem might not have a solution within the desired setting. It may be impossible for a deaf child to

succeed in an integrated setting no matter what services you can get for him. The solution might be to send him to a residential school, although you may not like that solution.

8. It is possible to win the battle and lose the war. Forcing an unwanted solution on a teacher can backfire. The professionals can make the solution fail—consciously or unconsciously—if they do not feel that they had some choice in the solution of a problem.

9. When a problem really cannot be resolved, don't continue struggling alone, especially if you are trying to change the basic structure of the system. *Get help.*

10. Long before problems develop, show your support of the agency and professionals involved, through a note of thanks, a comment about an interesting bulletin board, etc.

11. Don't accept excuses. Be suspicious when you are always told that everything is just fine, or that your child is the only problem in the school. The truth is usually someplace in between.

OTHER SUGGESTIONS

There are several sources of further information on parent groups and activism (Baker, 1976; Biklen, 1974). Roberta Thomas (personal communication, 1980) has provided some ideas about how to deal with more serious situations in which there are fundamental disagreements. We summarize her remarks here. Parents can change professionals or schools, which is not always possible or practical, or they can try to change their minds or policies. Before trying to change minds and policies (". . . a lot of hard, exhausting, frustrating work"), Thomas suggests writing down in detail why you believe your child needs what you think he needs. You should get help from all possible sources. Join a parent group or organize a chapter of the IAPD to have the force of numbers behind you and to raise funds that may be necessary. Affiliate with influential deaf persons and other parent groups serving other disabilities, if appropriate. Have representation from the deaf community and access to a professional who shares your beliefs. A lawyer is very helpful and sometimes essential. Develop your program with the guiding principle of always seeking to negotiate, persuade, and educate before trying pressure tactics. Find out *who* must be influenced, and seek an interview. Send a letter afterwards. If you get no satisfaction, it may be necessary to consider letter-writing campaigns, public hearings, radio and TV interviews, newspaper articles, political pressure, and legal avenues, but these are a last resort.

Factually wrong statements from a professional or administrator who has influence over your child's life or education should raise doubts about that person's competence *in the field of deafness*. Examples of faulty ideas are: 1) deaf children's needs are no different from those of all hearing-impaired children; 2) deaf children are naturally impulsive or limited in attainment; 3) a deaf child's behavior problems are always caused by brain damage; 4) amplification is useless for all profoundly deaf children; 5) sign languages are not true languages—they have no grammar, convey only concrete information, and will prevent the development of speech; and 6) most intelligent deaf children with cooperative parents can function fully in "the hearing world" and will not need to associate with other deaf people.

WHAT ARE THE CHARACTERISTICS OF A "GOOD" PROFESSIONAL?

The emphasis upon potentially adversarial relationships does not mean that most or many encounters between parents and professionals will be negative. Some professional qualities that are valued are:

1. Seeing people as individuals; interest in you and your child's ideas and feelings.
2. Availability and dependability.
3. Honesty about personal limitations and mistakes.

4. Willingness to change opinion when presented with new facts.
5. Ability to explain decisions, policies, and technical terms.

CONCLUSIONS

Parents and professionals sometimes have different views because they have different priorities, experiences, and sources of information. Problem-solving requires that both parties recognize this fact. In the presence of enough good will, many potential problems can be settled so that the feeling of partnership can be sustained. At other times, the fundamental nature of the disagreement cannot be resolved by parents without recourse to activism or by professionals without authoritarianism.

Many important changes have been brought about by parent groups. The present climate of increasing parent participation in planning offers positive opportunities, but also presents the possibility of frustration with rising expectations.

SUMMARY

1. Parents and professionals share the basic goal of
    helping deaf children to achieve the most they
    can. Many factors make it difficult to maintain a
    focus on this goal: differing priorities and levels of
    knowledge about deafness, gaps in information
    about the child, assumptions, personality styles,
    past experiences, pressures from elsewhere, and
    not understanding the system.
2. Parents who feel they need to obtain services
    from someone who disagrees with them should
    try to avoid making threats or acting impulsively.
    It may be helpful to clarify your thinking, to
    discuss the issue with others, and to form or join
    parent groups. Linkage with deaf people and
    professionals who share common ideas on
    significant matters is always a good idea.
3. There are many possible sources of dispute;
    action is more likely to be successful if the
    reasons are understood and simple solutions are
    tried first.
4. Good record-keeping is basic.
5. Professionals cannot be expert in everything, but
    their position may encourage them to act as if
    they are.
6. Some suggestions are made for creating change
    when the simpler techniques fail.

Chapter 20

INTERPRETERS

INTRODUCTION

Interpreters play an important part in relationships between hearing and deaf persons, and although the majority of their work has been with adults, services for children and teenagers are becoming more important.

This chapter presents a very brief picture of interpreting. Much more information can be obtained from an introductory book on interpreting, edited by Caccamise and his co-workers (1980) and published by the Registry of Interpreters for the Deaf. Other useful resources are Caccamise et al. (1978) and Ingram and Ingram (1977).

Because the field of interpreting is developing rapidly, we suggest that you familiarize yourself with your local services through appropriate organizations.

WHAT IS INTERPRETING?

An interpreter conveys one person's message to another, which involves a change in *language* (for example, between ASL or BSL and spoken or written English), or in *mode* (between signed English and spoken or written English). Technically, the use of the term "interpreting" should be restricted to a change in *language*, and the term "transliterating" should be used for a change in *mode*. ("Translating" refers to the conversion of one written language to another.) Ordinarily the first two types of language conversion are classed together. This looseness of terminology should not obscure the fact that transliterating skills between a sign code and English are not sufficient for many deaf persons.

Oral interpreters clearly, but inaudibly, mouth the words said by a speaker and may change a few words that are difficult to speechread (Northcott, 1979). This can be helpful, because in many situations speechreading is difficult even for those with good English. In *simultaneous interpreting*, the interpreter mouths *and* signs everything that the speaker is saying, whereas in *manual interpreting* not everything is mouthed (especially when sign language, as distinct from a sign code, is used). Finally, *voice interpreting* involves speaking what the deaf person is signing (this is the same as the old term *reverse interpreting*).

The skills and needs of the persons present determine the kinds of interpreting necessary. The interpreter seeks to convey the *entire* message, including the mood and attitude of the communicators, without imposing his or her own views or feelings. A British survey showed that accuracy of communication is more important to deaf people than speed (Kyle, Jones, and Woll, 1979).

WHAT HAPPENED IN THE PAST?

Before the recent efforts to promote interpreting as a profession, those serving as interpreters were likely to be hearing persons with deaf parents; clergymen working with deaf people; or social workers, teachers, or parents who had acquired some proficiency in signing. Their abilities varied widely and there was no assurance of competency, even in matters as important as legal proceedings. Even a person who knew both languages may not have been capable of interpreting; the same could be true with two spoken languages. If the deaf person was using a native sign language, many interpreters could not convey the meaning in English. Conflicts of interest with relatives or with others acting as interpreters sometimes occurred (this is still possible).

THE RISE OF PROFESSIONAL INTERPRETING

The Registry of Interpreters for the Deaf (RID) was founded in the United States in 1964 and incorporated in 1972. Similar efforts have also been under way in Canada, Australia, Scandinavia, and Britain. University degrees are now awarded in the interpreting field.

There are several reasons why training, certification, a registry, and a code of ethics are necessary for the interpreting field. Two reasons are illustrated by the following vignettes:

> A deaf teenage girl was interviewed by a psychiatrist. Her mother acted as interpreter, claiming that she knew sign language and had no communication problem. An observer who was familiar with signing recognized that the mother was using "home signs" rather than sign language or a sign code. Her daughter did know ASL and PSE, but these skills could not be utilized in the interview.

> The parents of a deaf woman died. During the reading of the will her sister acted as interpreter but did not inform her of her right to challenge the distribution of her parents' assets among the children. She only discovered this later and, with a qualified interpreter, successfully fought for her legal rights.

In the first instance, the psychiatrist could not know whether the communications from his patient were her own or her mother's, which could seriously affect his judgment. In the second case, there was a conflict of interest in addition to possible communication problems. In court situations, judges who are unfamiliar with interpreting may require a word-for-sign literal rendering of all communication, which seriously penalizes any deaf person who is without adequate English skills. In some cases, the civil rights of deaf persons are at issue regarding the availability and quality of interpreting. Finally, there has been a great increase in the demand for interpreters for educational, medical, mental health, legal, and rehabilitation settings (as well as for deaf-blind persons), positions that require special training and experience as well as great discretion and awareness of the need for confidentiality. [For example, court and medical interpreters need to know the signs for sexual behavior and drug use (Woodward, 1979, 1980).]

CODE OF ETHICS

Codes of ethics for interpreters have been developed for very good reasons. The deaf community is relatively small and personal information is communicated remarkably rapidly. Concern over the manner in which sensitive matters are revealed is therefore only natural. If the interpreter is working only on behalf of one deaf person (for example in a physician's office) there is often an expectation by the inexperienced hearing person that the interpreter will act as counselor or will reveal other information about the deaf individual that is not part of the interpreter's mandate. If such additional information is given, the interpreter's impartiality as a facilitator of communication is lost.

Here are some of the general guidelines of the RID Code (note that where "interpreter" is stated, "transliterator" is equally appropriate):

1. Interpreters shall keep all assignment-related information strictly confidential.
2. Interpreters shall render the message faithfully, always conveying the content of the message and the spirit of the speaker, using language most readily understood by the person(s) whom they serve.
3. Interpreters shall not counsel or advise those whom they serve, or interject personal opinions.
4. Interpreters shall accept assignments using discretion with regard to skill, setting, and the consumers involved.
5. Interpreters shall request compensation for services in a professional and judicious manner.
6. Interpreters shall function in a manner appropriate to the situation.

Also of concern are the continued education of interpreters and the maintenance of high standards within the profession (Caccamise et al., 1980).

CERTIFICATION

A certification board (usually with a majority of hearing-impaired members) examines interpreter candidates, who are required to interpret and transliterate in a variety of situations and at several levels of language complexity. Different skill levels are recognized in the certification. The registry enables courts, schools, or other organizations or individuals to obtain competent services.

POSITIVE EFFECTS OF INTERPRETER AVAILABILITY

Owens (personal communication, 1980) describes how improved availability and skills of interpreters brought about a changed awareness of, and attitude toward, deafness and deaf people. She notes that colleges are now more willing to establish interpreter training programs and to provide them for deaf students. "The role of the interpreter is one of the most vital in the life of a deaf person . . . Parents should be strong supporters of any program that will teach, screen, and certify interpreters for the future well-being of their family and especially their deaf child." Thomas (personal communication, 1980) emphasizes that deaf children should learn how to use interpreters early in life, because it will increase their independence.

Another important benefit of having interpreters available is the great increase in the numbers of deaf people attending trade schools, colleges, and universities with interpreter services.

LIMITATIONS

Interpreters cannot solve all communication problems. They cannot make up for a student's lack of preparation for a class. Nor can they ensure that a physician gives an explanation in language that the *interpreter* can understand and convey. Newman comments (personal communication, 1980):

> Understanding an interpreter depends upon the degree of language sophistication of the child. Our attention tends to stray when information comes from an interpreter rather than from "the horse's mouth." Parents should understand clearly the risks and limitations of having an interpreter with mainstreamed children, as well as the benefits. My own deaf child could not understand her interpreter.

Because deaf people are so variable in their language skills, interpreters must be able to make large adjustments. A series of different interpreters on different days may not work out well, even if all are certified. There are advantages if the teacher can sign and if hearing classmates learn basic signs and fingerspelling.

When the subject being interpreted is complicated, deaf people are very dependent upon good interpreting skills. If a particular interpreter is not satisfactory, it may be very awkward to demand a change. This is one reason why consultation ahead of time may be important when a choice of interpreters is available.

Interpreting is tiring work. When the demands are heavy and last long, more than one interpreter is necessary so that they may take turns.

In some cases two kinds of interpreting may be required simultaneously: two spoken languages may be involved, or the deaf person's signing skills may seem so poor that a deaf native signer may need to help the interpreter.

Many deaf people learn to fake understanding because they do not want the nuisance of frequently requesting clarification. Interpreters need to check to see that the message received is being understood.

COSTS

Interpreters may work full-time or part-time, or they may free-lance. In some areas interpreting services are free, and are paid by an agency; in others, fees may be charged.

PARENTS' AND PROFESSIONALS' RESPONSIBILITIES

Parents of deaf children who have some signing skills should refuse to serve as interpreters when it is against the best interests of the deaf people concerned. A certified interpreter should be demanded. If this is impossible, interpretation should be done only with a clear explanation of the reasons for using a non-professional and of the limitations involved. Similarly, parents should refuse to interpret for their own children in certain important situations. Physicians, lawyers, or others working with deaf persons should press for a competent interpreter. This type of insistence has two benefits: better communication for the deaf person immediately concerned, and the establishment (or further development) of a group of trained interpreters because of legitimate need.

CONCLUSIONS

Interpreting is a new field that is being increasingly professionalized and specialized. With the move toward integration and the more frequent attendance of deaf people at colleges and universities, it can be expected that more interpreter services will be required. There is still much to be learned about the most efficient ways to train and use interpreters. Although better skills are now available, deaf people still have an obligation to express dissatisfaction when they receive services that do not meet their needs.

SUMMARY

1. Interpreting is the facilitation of communication between two or more people who cannot otherwise understand each other. This may involve a change of language or of mode.
2. Differences between oral, simultaneous, manual, and voice interpreting are described.
3. Training, certification, and the establishment of registries are relatively new developments. Confidentiality and not intruding with personal judgments and feelings are important considerations for interpreters.
4. In addition to benefits, there are limitations to interpreting. It may be arduous, complicated work, and it does not always ensure that the desired comprehension will be achieved.
5. Deaf children should learn how to use an interpreter. In integrated or mainstreamed settings interpreters may be essential, but some parents and deaf persons prefer that the teacher sign and that classmates learn at least basic signs and fingerspelling.

Chapter 21

TECHNICAL AIDS

INTRODUCTION

Let's follow the actions of a deaf teenager, Jeff Jones, as he makes a telephone call. He wants to discuss plans for the weekend with his deaf friend, Bob Smith, who lives across the city. Before his and Bob's parents got them TDDs (Telecommunication Device for the Deaf), others would have to relay messages for the boys. This posed a problem, because Jeff's parents are both deaf.

Jeff dials the number and then places his telephone handset on the TDD. He can see the pattern of Bob's phone ringing, and can distinguish this from a busy signal, because a small light flashes in time with the sound of the ringing. The light stops flashing, so Jeff assumes someone has picked up the phone. Actually Bob has put his handset on his TDD. He types "BOB HERE GA" (meaning "Go Ahead"). Jeff types "HI THIS IS JEFF . . ." and continues the message, alternating turns with Bob by typing "GA." As the end of the conversation approaches, Jeff says "OK WILL MEET YOU THERE AT SEVEN GA TO SK." This tells Bob that Jeff is finished unless Bob wishes to add something. He types "FINE SEE YOU LATER SKSK" (meaning "Stop Keying") and Jeff terminates with his own "SKSK" and both hang up.

If Mrs. Smith had answered the phone, she would have said "Hello" by voice. If there were no reply, she would assume that a deaf person was calling and would use the TDD. If Bob were in the house alone, he would connect his signaling device, which would flash a light when the phone rang. If it were a hearing person calling by voice, no conversation would have been possible.

The details of such a scene vary somewhat with the type of TDD, but the situation illustrates how technical aids have reduced the practical problems of being deaf. There are other tasks that deaf people accomplish: waking up on time, answering the doorbell, recognizing a baby's cry, and enjoying television. Many of these situations have been transformed by modern technology for the benefit of deaf people, but the techniques and equipment may not yet be available in all areas. A complete presentation of all the developments is impossible here, but parent groups or groups of deaf people in your area will know what is available to you.

TELEPHONE (TDD)

A few deaf persons and many hard-of-hearing persons can use telephones with amplifiers or can place special coils in their hearing aids. For most of the children we are discussing, however, voice communication on the telephone is not possible. For them, there are now many kinds of devices available in some parts of the world to communicate letters and numbers rather than voice. (Some of these aids are shown in Figure 11.) Although communication devices were originally known in North America as "TTYs" (teletypewriters), the preferred new designation is "TDD" (Telecommunication Device for the Deaf). All devices operate on the basic principle of converting typed letters, numbers, and punctuation marks into a tone signal that is sent through the ordinary telephone handset and phone lines and decoded by a compatible TDD at the receiving end. The display may be on paper (*hard copy*), on a lighted read-out similar to an electronic calculator, or both. Many (but not all) devices are compatible with each other. Long-distance and international calls can be made, especially now that direct dialing is more widespread.

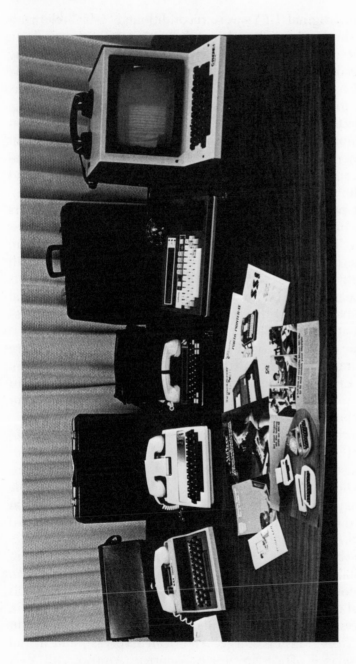

Figure 11. Examples of North American telecommunication devices for the deaf (TDDs). [Courtesy of Gordon J. K. Gell and Children's Hospital, through the Western Institute for the Deaf.]

The original TTYs were reconditioned "5-bit" teleprinters of the kind employed by telegraph companies, with an acoustic coupler (invented by a deaf physicist) for coding and decoding. This type of device is usually donated and gives a hard copy of the conversation, but is non-portable, is noisy for hearing neighbors, and requires frequent servicing.

Electronic miniaturization has led to the modern portables shown in Figure 11. There are many new options that have increased the usefulness of the TDD: answering machines, special radio programs giving news and weather, and a Braille adaptation for those who are deaf and blind.

At present, "8-bit" systems for linkage with computers are being developed that are *not* compatible with most existing TDDs. Some devices can operate on either system, but there are still problems to be worked out in North America in the next few years. Telephone developments have been reviewed by Castle (1979). There is an annual international TDD directory that also has a "yellow pages" section advertising all the TDD types in North America.

One disadvantage of the TDD system is that calls require more time than voice calls and may therefore be much more costly. Efforts are being made, with some success, to obtain special rates for deaf people in some American states and in other countries.

Portable machines may cost from $180 to more than $600 (U.S.A.). By 1983, California telephone companies must install TDDs at the same cost as regular telephones. Saskatchewan provides free TDDs, and in British Columbia they may be obtained on a lease-purchase arrangement at reduced cost through the Western Institute for the Deaf. In the U.S.A., TDDs are tax-deductible.

In the past few years there has been a rapid increase in the installation of TDD services in police stations, hospitals, crisis centers, government offices, department stores, schools for deaf children, airline offices (National Airlines in Miami), in hotels with toll-free numbers (Holiday Inns), in credit card offices (MasterCharge, American Express), and in rail travel service offices in North America (Amtrak and VIA

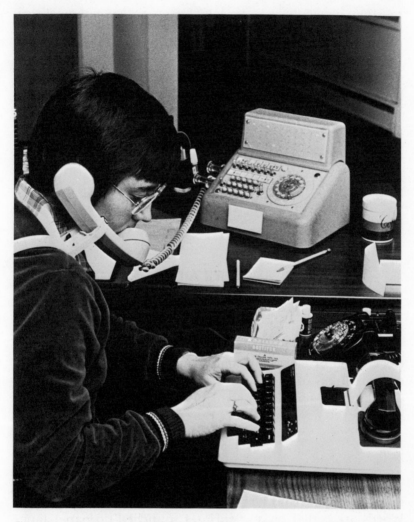

Figure 12.   Message center for TDD users. [Courtesy of Gordon J. K. Gell and Children's Hospital, through the Western Institute for the Deaf.]

Rail). Some U.S. Congressmen can be called by their deaf constituents. Starting in June 1980 the Bell Telephone System in the U.S.A. offered nationwide 24-hour toll-free TDD Operator Services. This enables deaf TDD owners to make credit-card, collect, person-to-person, and service calls.

Long-distance calls can be billed to a third number. These impressive new services are described in a customer information booklet for Bell subscribers.

An agency serving the deaf community may provide a message service for TDD users, such as changing physician appointments or notifying employers of illness (see Figure 12). The Western Institute for the Deaf has a recorded message for deaf callers that relates any announcements or important recreational news.

The principle benefit of TDDs is that they offer deaf children and teenagers the opportunity to expand their social relationships and thereby increase the motivation to improve their English.

OTHER AIDS

Wake-up Alarms

To provide a wake-up alarm for a deaf person, an ordinary clock radio or electronic alarm can be adapted to flash one or more lights or to activate a small vibrator under a mattress or pillow. Alarm clocks can thus be as much of a help (or nuisance) to deaf persons as they are to hearing people.

Radio

The Pennsylvania School for the Deaf in Philadelphia has the world's first and largest radio network for deaf people. Words are coded on a teleprinter, punched on paper tape, then converted into audible tones that are sent via telephone to Temple University's FM station. There the tones are broadcast within a 30-mile to 50-mile radius. Specially tuned home radio receivers are connected with TDDs for the print-out of news. (In a sense this is "captioned radio.") There are over 600 free radio receivers in use, provided by a grant from the Nevil Foundation (*Deaf American* May 1980, 32(9):37).

Doorbell

The doorbell button can be connected with lights that flash on and off at a rate recognizably different from other devices in the same home (such as the telephone signaler). A knock on the door (without an electronic button) can also be displayed. Deaf-blind persons may use a combination of a fan and vibrating box. There are also combinations that include a telephone signaler, doorbell, wake-up alarm, baby-cry device, and burglar alarm.

Baby-Cry Device

With the installation of a baby-cry device, a microphone in the baby's room converts the cry into a light or vibration pattern, which is easily distinguished from a telephone or doorbell signal. (The deaf person "sees" what the hearing person "hears.")

Smoke Alarms, Burglar Alarms

Alerting devices to detect smoke and burglary can be attached to standard light or vibration alarms.

Captioned Films

Deaf people have always been interested in films that they can understand. Foreign films with subtitles have been popular. Some deaf clubs show specially captioned films. Recently the first full-feature film was made using ASL and voice—it's called "Think Me Nothing."

Television

Television programs specifically serving the deaf community have been produced in recent years. Some areas have programs of local interest. Occasionally there are nationally broadcast religious or cultural shows (a recent example in

North America was Dylan Thomas' "A Child's Christmas in Wales," produced by the National Theater of the Deaf). Nevertheless, most TV programs cannot be enjoyed by deaf people, and constant requests to a hearing viewer to interpret what is happening are disruptive and impractical. A recent solution is the optional *line 21 closed captioning* in the U.S.A., in which a decoding device (sold only by Sears, Roebuck, and Co.) displays captions on the bottom of the TV screen. These captions are not seen by hearing viewers in homes without the decoder. The captions are prepared by the National Captioning Institute and provide approximately 20 hours a week of captioned viewing (1980 estimate). Incentives and legal requirements are being worked out to ensure that TV stations use this system.

Systems of access to computer banks via telephones and TV screens are being developed for the general population and will be useful to deaf people. In Britain both the BBC and ITV provide instant news, weather, and other information with a decoder or a modified TV set.

Battery Chargers

Devices to test and recharge batteries for hearing aids are now available in North America.

Pets

Although they are not strictly "technical aids," deaf people find that dogs are useful as more than just companions: they can alert you to someone at the door and can do even more with special training. (Dogs can learn to respond to simple signs as well as to spoken commands.)

CONCLUSIONS

We have presented a few of the important technical advances that have made deaf people's lives easier in the last few years and that hold promise for even better things to come. Because of inflation and rapid technological advances, it is advisable to check with your local or national organizations for the latest information on these devices. The IAPD newsletter *The Endeavor*, the *Deaf American*, the *Deaf Canadian*, *Hearing*, *Talk*, and the *British Deaf News* are examples of good sources. Detailed information about TDD developments in North America can be obtained from Telecommunication Devices for the Deaf, Inc., 814 Thayer Ave., Silver Spring, Maryland 20910.

SUMMARY

1. Several communication devices are briefly
    described that enable deaf persons to use alarm
    clocks, doorbells, telephones, burglar and smoke
    alarms, television, radio, and films.
2. Existing devices can alert a deaf person to a baby
    crying or to someone knocking on the door.
3. New legislation, as well as voluntary compliance,
    have resulted in the rapid spread of
    telecommunication device services throughout
    North America.

Chapter 22

DEAF CHILDREN WITH OTHER DISABILITIES

... this strange, normal-looking but hiddenly complicated little boy ... [Browning, 1972, p. 84]

INTRODUCTION

The combination of each child's disabilities with his or her personality, intelligence, temperament, and upbringing produces a unique situation. Intervention programs are few, and those that do exist are costly. Although there are many reports of substantial progress with individual children or groups of children, there are few long-term follow-up or comparative studies.

In this chapter, we outline some of the difficulties in assessment and program development, briefly describe some of the more common combinations of disabilities, and indicate sources of further reading, because we can discuss this complicated subject only briefly here.

There are several useful general references on the subject of multiply disabled deaf children: Haag (1978), Power and Quigley (1971), Schein (1974, 1975, 1979a), Shroyer and Tweedie (1979), Stewart (1974, 1978), and Vernon (1969).

WHO ARE THE DEAF CHILDREN WITH MULTIPLE DISABILITIES?

In Chapter 7, a distinction was made among the terms "impairment," "disability," and "handicap." It is important

291

to keep these differences in mind. Perhaps everyone has at least some degree of impairment in one or more areas of functioning, but for most of us this disability is not significant. Many deaf children also have one or more additional impairments, but these might not interfere with any important areas of functioning.

The Office of Demographic Studies of Gallaudet College runs an annual survey of American hearing-impaired students. Consistently high rates of additional disabilities are reported, but this rate (usually about one-third of all hearing-impaired students) is based upon highly variable teacher reports. When a careful study is done of groups of deaf children and when definitions of additional disabilities are agreed upon, the rate of additional disability is much lower, but still significant. Lennan (1979) has pointed out that when teachers are asked their definitions of a category of additional disability (such as mental retardation), there is very little agreement.

Conrad (1979) has criticized the figures in Gallaudet's American survey:

> . . . of all factors which might be relevant to academic achievement by the deaf, that factor loosely described as "additional handicaps" is most misleading, confused, and unreliable. Yet it is one which is perhaps cited more than any other by teachers to account for poor school performance. [p. 59]

Using more strict standards of testing, Conrad found an overall rate of 11% with additional disabilities; the rate was higher in boys than in girls, and higher in non-hereditary than in hereditary deafness. (These differences have been confirmed by other investigators.) Conrad felt that the most "suspicious" categories (those not well defined) were emotional or behavior problems, and "brain damage."

Stewart (1974) strongly criticized the confused labeling of multiply handicapped deaf individuals. He pointed out that one *disability* (hearing) might lead to multiple *handicaps* (problems in speech, reading, social maturity), while several *disabilities* (such as deafness plus loss of a leg) might *not* produce multiple handicaps.

There are also other labels (besides the two mentioned by Conrad) that tend to be loosely used. A word of caution is needed at this point: one of these labels may be applied to your own child by a physician or psychologist. We have no desire to create antagonism between parents and professionals, nor are we saying that these labels *never* should be applied. It is a matter of demonstrating *care* in using them, because the behavior on which the diagnosis is based may have other causes.

TYPES OF ADDITIONAL DISABILITIES

Mental Retardation

The usual definition of mental retardation is an IQ (*intelligence quotient*) of 70 or less, accompanied by problems in adaptive behavior. The figure of 3% is usually quoted for the proportion of retarded individuals in the general population. Among deaf people, the rate is higher (8%–12%) because of overlap in the causes of both conditions.

The IQ range from 50 to 70 is sometimes referred to as "educable mental retardation," and the 30 to 50 range is termed "trainable," implying that those persons falling in that range are unlikely to learn school subjects, such as reading, with comprehension. (This dividing line is not absolute, however.)

Assessment of mental retardation is difficult in the presence of deafness, and some deaf children with normal or close-to-normal intelligence are misclassified as retarded either because those testing them cannot communicate with them or because the children's behavior is not understood. In some cases, the deafness has not yet been identified (Denmark, 1978).

Traditionally, if deaf mentally retarded children were in any program, it would be in a special class in a school for the deaf or in a residential facility for mentally retarded children. There have been relatively few special programs of this type, and rarely has the staff had the necessary specialized training.

The combination of deafness with mental retardation tends to produce severe deficiencies in life experience. A structured program with clearly established developmental objectives that are regularly revised has been found to be helpful (Tweedie and Shroyer, 1979).

There are four areas for possible communication development: speech, manual, graphic (reading, writing), and special symbol systems (such as Blissymbolics). Very few children can make much use of speech communication unless there is a substantial remnant of hearing for speech. As with manual communication, a full sign language or sign code is often too complex (Fristoe and Lloyd, 1978). Simplified systems have been developed in the United Kingdom (Cornforth, Johnston, and Walker, 1976), and North American usage has been reviewed by Fristoe and Lloyd (1978), Goodman, Wilson, and Bornstein (1978), and Wilbur (1979). (Sign codes are being used for mentally retarded children with normal hearing who have language difficulties.) The graphic mode is usually not very useful; this includes fingerspelling. Several invented symbol systems are in use, and are described by Schiefelbusch (1980), Tweedie and Shroyer (1979), and Vanderheiden and Grilley (1977).

It is especially important for parents to know that the label "mental retardation," even if accurate, covers a wide range of abilities. The public image of mental retardation is rarely correct. Many persons believe that it refers to a person who is helpless or who can develop no self-care skills, and who will learn nothing. In reality, many mentally retarded persons become productive members of society. However, in order for deaf persons with reduced general intelligence to make the most of their abilities, special assistance is needed.

Naiman (1979) described an extensive program for hearing-impaired retarded adolescents in a local New York City school. Most children made considerable progress, some enough to integrate into a regular class for deaf children. Naiman concluded that deaf retarded children are very different from each other and that no one type of program could possibly meet all their needs. She advocated a range of settings, services, and models of acceptable social behavior.

McCormack's 1978 book is a good exposition of the problems and feelings of parents of retarded children.

Cerebral Palsy

Cerebral palsy is not a disease. It is a description of a group of conditions caused by damage to the parts of the brain controlling movement. The condition may be so mild that the child is only slightly clumsy, or it may be severe enough that the affected person cannot speak, walk, or even swallow properly. There may be *spasticity,* in which some of the muscles are too tight; *athetosis,* in which there are writhing, involuntary movements; *ataxia,* in which there are severe balance problems; *atonia,* in which there is poor muscle tone; or combinations of all of these. Areas of the brain other than those controlling movement may be affected: there is a higher rate in those with cerebral palsy than in the general population of mental retardation, seizures, and language problems, but most cerebral-palsied children are not affected in these additional ways.

Cunningham and Holt (1977) studied ten English children with deafness and cerebral palsy. There were delays in both diagnoses of from 1 to 3½ years. *All* were misdiagnosed as mentally retarded in the first year of life; deafness was usually identified later than the cerebral palsy.

> The diagnosis of retardation in the first year of life should be made with the greatest of care and caution and, even if suspected, should be followed by referral to a consultant paediatrician, thorough investigation, and the initiation of developmental guidance and surveillance. [p. 482]

Four of the ten children in the English study had some useful speech; the others had so much involvement of the muscles used in speech that this skill was deemed impossible to train. *All* of the children had enough hand control for

gestures and sign language (although this was being taught
to only one child, with rapid progress). Problems in diagnosis
were caused by failure to respond to various tests at the
expected age, poor head control, and involuntary responses.

Deaf children with cerebral palsy need expert help in at
least two areas: physical management (such as mobility and
physiotherapy) and communication. Most schools for physically handicapped children do not provide for deaf students
(noise levels may be extremely high, for example). The
physically handicapped child may also have difficulties in
some schools for deaf children (architectural barriers). Special training of teachers and close coordination of services
are highly desirable because of special learning problems.

Fitch (1972) described an 11-year-old girl with cerebral
palsy who had been misdiagnosed as retarded and recommended for institutional placement. When a communication
program was started, she learned signs and fingerspelling
rapidly: in eight months she had mastered a vocabulary of
more than 500 signs, a reading vocabulary of over 100
words, and basic arithmetic processes. Once communication
was well established, better testing of her hearing was possible. Her true potential had previously been impossible to
assess. Fitch concludes:

> Careful consideration should be given to the severely involved child whose past
> records indicate little hope of progress. It is entirely possible that the next eval-
> uation may reveal some clue to a communication process that may completely
> change previous prognosis. [p. 378]

Fenn and Rowe (1975) used simplified Paget-Gorman
signs with non-communicating retarded cerebral-palsied
children, many of whom were deaf. Results were encouraging, and in some children speech improved.

General references that are useful for parents are Blencowe (1969) and Finnie (1975).

Visual Impairment

Most children who are loosely labeled "deaf-blind" are not
totally deaf and totally blind. McInnes and Treffry (1977)

stated:

> . . . the deaf-blind child is not a deaf child who cannot see, a blind child who cannot hear, nor a retarded child with visual and auditory problems. He is a child with a multiplicity of problems. It may be of use to the medical profession to identify major handicaps . . . However useful this information is in terms of medical treatment, it can be misleading—even damaging—in terms of programming for the deaf-blind child. If the deaf-blind child must be identified as having a major handicap, then that major handicap should be identified as *multi-sensory deprivation* (MSD). [p. 337]

We use the MSD abbreviation in this book.

American legislation defines a "deaf-blind" child educationally, rather than medically. Such a child has both auditory and visual disabilities, the combination of which causes such severe communication and other developmental and educational problems that he cannot properly be accommodated in special education programs either for the visually or hearing-impaired child (Hammer, 1973). MSD children with later onset of their multiple disabilities have different problems than those whose disabilities start at (or shortly after) birth. One of the major difficulties is that with very 'early onset of MSD and impairment of both distance senses (vision and hearing), the children may require intensive intervention before they express any desire to communicate with others (Hammer, 1973).

Vernon, Bair, and Lotz (1979) reviewed psychological evaluation of MSD children. There are no standardized tests. Psychological findings should be combined with a careful history (including information about the cause), a checklist of skills, and a record of observed progress in a program.

Klein (1978) emphasized the following bases for program development: 1) early identification; 2) parent involvement; 3) an individualized, developmentally based, optimistic approach; 4) cooperation of several professional disciplines; and 5) support and periodic relief for parents.

Hicks and Pfau (1979) surveyed the frequency of the occurrence of visual impairment in the United States and the services available to treat it. Depending upon the type of test and the definitions used, the rate of visual problems in deaf children ranged from 8% to 50%. These of course included refractive errors (minor visual problems requiring glasses) as well as severe handicaps. *Deaf children are more likely than hearing children to have or to develop visual problems, and they are much more dependent upon good vision.*

Tibbenham, Peckham, and Gardiner (1978) have reported extensive follow-up studies of vision in British children. Tests were performed at ages seven, eleven, and sixteen. Many children who were found to be normal at one of these ages had defective vision at a later examination. For example, 18% of those reported as normal at age seven (and 12% of those normal at age eleven) had defects at age sixteen. *These results clearly demonstrate that regular vision testing is important for all children.*

MSD children need, above all, to develop a communication system. Jensema (1979) has argued that there is a great need for careful assessment before a particular language system is selected for an MSD child. If there is sufficient vision, signs may be useful; there are other slower methods if enough vision is not present.

Usher's syndrome presents special problems. This is a hereditary (recessive) condition that starts with profound congenital deafness. Later there is gradual loss of vision, often to the point of complete blindness, although there are great differences in the age of onset and the rate of visual loss. Reduction in night vision is first noted, then loss of peripheral vision (what you see away from the line of focus), and finally weakened central vision. Usher's syndrome is one form of *retinitis pigmentosa*, in which pigment (colored material) is deposited in, and damages, the light-sensitive portion of the eye (retina).

Usher's syndrome accounts for about half of all deaf-blindness in adults and probably affects about 3%–6% of all congenitally deaf children. The frequency in the general population is reported to be only three per 100,000.

Although there is no treatment available, regular examinations by an ophthalmologist (eye doctor) are recommended for all deaf children and can help to identify Usher's syndrome in its early stages. Genetic counseling is important to enable families to prevent future pregnancies if they so wish. It is also important for the affected children or adults to understand what is happening to them. They should avoid training for a job that will be impossible to perform without vision. Individual, family, and group counseling may assist adjustment.

The National Retinitis Pigmentosa Foundation (see Resource List) was founded by parents in the United States in 1971 and now has 55 chapters in five countries; it has provided much useful information and millions of dollars for research.

We mention this condition because we feel it must be described as part of the problem of multiple disabilities. Some parents may be unnecessarily frightened when they learn about it. Do not assume that your child may be going blind if he or she occasionally knocks into things at night. Deaf children have poorer balance than hearing children, and balance is always worse in the dark (Lindsey and O'Neal, 1976).

An entire issue of the *American Annals of the Deaf* (English, 1978) was devoted to Usher's syndrome, including identification, child and family adjustment, and vocational training. Several reports and brochures have been published by the National Academy of Gallaudet College.

Rubella Syndrome

In the more general area of MSD, there have been several encouraging developments. *Rubella syndrome*, a major cause of MSD, is now preventable by rubella vaccine. (It has recently been learned that children with the rubella syndrome are more likely to develop diabetes and thyroid problems. They should have regular check-ups.) Legislation in the United States in 1968 authorized regional centers for assessment and service. By 1973 the centers had identified 5,300 children with rubella syndrome. The Helen Keller National Center for Deaf-Blind Youths and Adults (with three regional centers) was authorized by Congress in 1967 and set up a few years later in the New York City area. Parent organizations and less extensive facilities are being developed in other countries. This represents a growing awareness of the problem and the needs of these children (Hammer, 1973).

Chess and her co-workers (Chess et al., 1971) performed a landmark study of children with congenital rubella syndrome (birth defects from German measles). Starting in 1967, these researchers studied 243 children whose mothers had had rubella during the 1964 epidemic. Twenty percent had no defects at all, 30% had one defect, 20% had two defects, and 30% had more than two defects. Hearing loss was by far the most common impairment. The main purpose of the study was to look at the relationships among behavior, physical disability, and family adjustment. Almost half the children had no psychiatric disorder. As the number of areas of disability increased, so did the risk of psychiatric problems, but there was no characteristic *type* of behavior. (Psychiatric disorder was diagnosed in 42% of those with hearing impairment).

Neurologically damaged children showed more difficult temperamental patterns, such as greater irregularity of body functions (sleeping, feeding, toileting), less adaptability, greater withdrawal tendencies, and more intense reactions. This is of practical significance: the ability of workers to persist with a program for temperamentally difficult children may depend upon an understanding of the children's negative reactions. Parents need to realize that they are not usually at fault for their child's behavior, that it is likely to improve, and that they need sympathetic understanding of their own negative reactions. Some rubella children show what is called "tactile defensiveness:" they resist being held or cuddled. This can be very distressing to parents.

The study also reported an important finding about tested intelligence: the children tended to improve with time. Some moved from the retarded into the normal range of tested IQ. Early test results are therefore not good predictors of later response. Program plans must be frequently revised.

(We have seen other rubella children who were "late bloomers," not only in IQ, but in relationship capacity and in behavior.)

Chess's research group has reported higher than expected rates of *childhood autism* among their children with rubella. There may have been differences in the types of epidemics, because in Vancouver (and in London, U.K.) this increase has not been found.

Hearing assessment in rubella children seems to be especially difficult; often there are inconsistencies from one audiogram to another, and a central language disorder may be suspected.

The measurement of head size is one way of determining whether a child is mentally retarded. Although most children with significant *microcephaly* (small heads) are indeed retarded, this is not true for all; some rubella children have small heads because their bodies are also small for their age.

Most important is for parents to be cautiously optimistic and to have the services of a professional team of workers who are open-minded about the child's future.

Two books on rubella syndrome have been published for parents (P. Freeman, 1975; Scott, Jan, and Freeman, 1977). There is also the autobiography of Smithdas, a well-known deaf-blind man (Smithdas, 1969); and Yoken (1979) has profiled the lives of nine deaf-blind adults. A guide for workers in deaf-blind residential settings has been edited by Lowell (1976). For parents and professionals, there is now a regular section on this subject in the *American Annals of the Deaf*, and Gallaudet College has established a special program. Cooperation between agencies serving hearing-impaired and visually impaired children and adults is increasing.

Aphasia, Dysphasia, or Central Language Disorder

There is probably no more confusing area of multiple disabilities than central language disorders. The original Greek meaning of the word "aphasia" is simply "without speech." Because most hearing children with this label have some speech, the term *dysphasia*, meaning impaired speech or language, is preferred. (Other terms used include "central language disorder," "central processing disorder," "auditory imperception," and "developmental aphasia.")

It is thought that hearing children with dysphasia "hear" sounds, but are not able to make sense of them or, if they can, they may not be able to put their response into words. There may be impairment in perception, discrimination of sounds, auditory memory, comprehension, word-finding, reading, and writing (Topp, 1977). Unlike in adult aphasia (which may occur after a stroke), there is *no* loss of previous functions; the children *fail to develop* normal language. Their condition may therefore be confused with mental retardation or emotional disturbance.

Sometimes deaf children are said to be aphasic or dysphasic. This is certainly much more difficult to diagnose in deaf than in hearing children, and conflicting professional opinions are not uncommon. We have seen some deaf children who were not making progress in oral-only programs wrongly labeled as "aphasic." It is also possible to wrongly suspect a central language problem in deaf children in a Total Communication program, when they fail to acquire signing skills for other reasons.

Because there are no clear-cut tests for developmental dysphasia, careful and repeated evaluations must be made, involving several disciplines: audiology, speech and language pathology, psychology, special education, and pediatrics. Sometimes pediatric neurology and child psychiatry must also be consulted. Parental observations are always helpful, and should include the child's use of non-verbal communication. The working plan developed by the team needs to be periodically revised. Other systems of communication may be necessary, or tasks may have to be broken down into smaller steps or be presented at a rate slower than the usual.

Some workers classify dysphasia in the more general category of *learning disability*. There are so many possible functions of the brain that can be impaired or inefficient that there is no complete list of disabilities and probably never will be. The best general advice that can be given is to take a careful look at all areas of the child's functioning (including physical, social, and psychological), and consult with the best and most flexible professionals available.

Browning (1972) has written an excellent book about the frustrations and satisfactions of a family with a hearing-impaired, dysphasic child, and Wyke (1978) has edited a technical review of this confusing field.

Psychiatric Disorder

Deaf children are somewhat more likely to have a disorder of behavior or emotions than are hearing children, but the causes of this fact are not well understood (Freeman, 1979). The use of the term "psychiatric disorder" does not mean that all these children need psychiatric care, or that only a psychiatrist can or should help. (A psychiatrist is a physician who specializes in disorders of feeling, thinking, and behavior. A psychologist, who is not a physician, has varied training in how people or animals behave, which may or may not include study of the treatment of behavior problems in children.) Because deaf children are likely to have so many different life experiences and limitations in our hearing society, we must be cautious about blaming problems on any one cause.

Naiman, Schein, and Stewart (1973) have made recommendations about deaf children who have serious behavior problems. Unfortunately, most day or residential schools for deaf children do not have adequate programs for these children or their families, nor do they have consultants who can communicate in signs. There is a great need for further program development in most parts of the world.

One diagnostic category that causes much confusion is so-called *hyperactivity* or *hyperkinetic impulse disorder*. Sometimes this is wrongly equated with learning disability or *minimal brain dysfunction* (MBD). In hyperactivity, the child is thought to be too active and to have a short attention span, to be impulsive and distractible, and to show poorly organized behavior. In recent years this has been elevated almost to the level of an epidemic in North America (although a much more conservative position is typical in the U.K.).

Studies have shown that about half of all children are described as overactive by their parents or teachers at one time or another. Rarely is there a direct *measurement* of the behavior. Many children so labeled are restless and learn poorly in school, but show no such behavior at home, where the expectations are different. A few children have consistently difficult behavior under all circumstances. Preschool-age normal children and children with *any* type of psychiatric disorder may be hyperactive—the behavior is not specific, and is not closely associated with brain damage. Poor communication, poor teaching or training, boredom, anxiety, and depression can also produce similar behavior. Shaffer and Greenhill (1979) have summarized this problem area very well. Beware of professionals or friends who tell you that they have a reliable way to identify or to treat such behavior problems; every type of treatment imaginable has been used, and claims of success have been made for each. Because hyperactivity does not represent a disease or a specific disorder, it is unlikely that there is one cause. Brain damage, lead poisoning, allergies, food additives, fluorescent lights, and many other factors have been indicted—but parents should be skeptical of claims that there is one single answer.

There are, of course, children with all sorts of problems, from specific impairments of brain function to difficult family situations, worries, poor schools, and unrecognized visual problems. There is no simple way to sort out these problems or to treat them. Thorough study is needed by people who can take the time to understand and communicate both with child and family.

Drug therapy has a definite place for certain "hyperactive" children, but should not be used as a substitute for a complete assessment.

Childhood autism is fortunately a rare disorder. The child may have a period of apparently normal development, but may fail to develop normal language. There is little or no warm relationship with other people and no emotional expression. There may be strange, repetitive rituals and insistence that things be just so. Many children avoid making eye contact, and typically they fail to reach out to be picked up or cuddled. Their parents may worry over the lack of social response. About half of autistic children are also mentally retarded, and some later develop seizures. Although it used to be thought that this failure of emotional and language development was caused by poor parenting, the evidence does not support this (Rutter and Schopler, 1978). (A neurological cause is suspected but has not been identified.) Children with dysphasia also show abnormal language use, but their relationships and behavior are much more normal (Bartak, Rutter, and Cox, 1975). Some autistic children are misdiagnosed as deaf because they tend to ignore sounds, particularly speech. Deaf children normally are visually observant and enjoy relationships. Sometimes a retarded deaf child or a rubella syndrome deaf child will start life showing little interest in people, and may then be confused with the truly autistic child who actively resists human social interaction. In those situations where bizarre behavior continues, a child psychiatrist should be consulted, and if there is question about hearing assessment, cooperation with the audiologist is advisable. There is no specific treatment for childhood autism, but educational programs have produced substantial changes in some autistic children, and some who are not deaf can use signs better than spoken words (Deich and Hodges, 1977; Fulweiler and Fouts, 1976).

Other Disabilities

We have not mentioned all additional disabilities (such as cardiac, epilepsy, orthopedic, or cleft palate) that may affect some deaf children. The emphasis upon medical labels should not lead us to ignore other factors, such as minority group and socioeconomic status. In some countries there is racial, religious, ethnic, financial, social class, or sex discrimination that may make services more difficult to obtain or that may affect choice of vocation. These factors may be more handicapping than some physical disabilities.

PROBLEMS OF ASSESSMENT

Personnel trained in deafness and additional disabilities are unfortunately scarce. The cooperation of several professionals is essential. The child ideally should be seen in more than one setting (home, school, office). An assessment in a clinic or hospital (unfamiliar surroundings) may not demonstrate the child's strengths. We prefer home and school visits (Freeman, 1967). It is particularly important to include in the assessment all those persons who know the child well and to look for sources of stress, boredom, and loneliness.

There is currently a welcome trend to include parents in conferences and to provide them with written reports. As a parent, it will probably help you to write down a list of your questions so they will not be forgotten; observations you have made that might not be repeated in a professional's office should also be noted. Once a plan is established, it should be regularly reviewed because it cannot be perfect.

It is generally easier to get a diagnosis than a program of action. Some professionals find it difficult to translate an evaluation into a program; this requires an experienced person who can set reasonable objectives. It may be helpful if the teacher or other person working with your child can accompany you to the assessments. Working with multiply handicapped deaf children is challenge enough without trying to cope with professional jealousies and territorial defenses. Try to find people who are not afraid to admit that they don't know everything.

FAMILY IMPLICATIONS

Meadow (1979) has described some of the problems parents face when their multiply disabled deaf child makes only slow progress. She suggested four areas in which parents might need help: 1) with external circumstances that could interfere with their efforts on behalf of their child (such as finances or housing); 2) with feelings, such as grief and anger; 3) with information about normal child development; and 4) with specific information about their child's unique situation.

One parent described how confusing it can be to try to relate diagnostic labels to everyday living:

It is not a case of not knowing the answers, but of not even knowing the questions to ask. The words—mongolism, retardation, brain damage—mean nothing in practical terms. They will tell you nothing about how the child will fit into the family, about sharing yourself between him and the rest of the family, about the ups and downs, the good days and the bad. [McCormack, 1978, pp. 18–19]

Parental reactions are likely to depend upon individual and marital strengths and weaknesses, the actual burden of care, the health of child and parents, the social network of friends and relatives, and professional support. Also important is the way in which professional recommendations are made and integrated. Periodic relief so that life has its lighter moments is essential.

Contact with other parents can be helpful, too. Other children in the family need attention, and a balance in meeting the needs of all family members is an ideal to strive for.

Finally, we present in a parent's own words why it is important to remain open-minded and patient, and how a teacher of the deaf can use ordinary life experiences to build a communication system:

We thought he was too sick and weak to learn. But we finally agreed to let the teacher come and visit with us. She was encouraging and said he just had to learn because he was so observant. I was skeptical. On her second visit she noticed that he had a hand motion that resembled the sign for "light." She immediately rushed to the light switch. That week the neighbours must have thought we were crazy with the lights blinking all the time. But he connected the hand motion with the result.

This child who had no verbal communication whatever,
acquired meaningful use of 286 signs over a 17-month
period and now uses sentences.

CONCLUSIONS

Multiply disabled deaf children are very different from each
other, and their unique needs must be evaluated and met in
usually less than ideal ways. There are still few trained
personnel, therefore much of the burden falls upon parents
and teachers. Much more could be done if schools were
convinced that many deaf children with multiple disabilities
have much greater potential than what is obvious or what
appears in test results. Perhaps schools could encourage
their funding bodies (usually governmental) to approve
additional training for their staff if the potential of these
children were recognized. Parent associations and professional groups also have a responsibility to make these points
clear to their schools and governments.

Because of the need for specialized training of teachers
and additional support staff, few local school districts (except
in the largest cities) can hope to satisfy parents who wish
their child to be served in their home community. Centralized
schools need to be retained as one important option.

We believe it would be helpful, especially in a time of
economic restrictions, if researchers and practitioners could
do better follow-up studies and could report the results of
giving multiply disabled deaf children a reasonable chance.

SUMMARY

1. Each multiply handicapped deaf child has special needs; labels tell us relatively little. No single program can be adequate for all.

2. The frequency of additional significant disabilities depends upon how statistical information is obtained and upon what definitions are used; the rate ranges from a conservative 11% to over one-third of all deaf children.

3. Assessment of deaf children who have multiple disabilities from birth is often difficult, and there are few fully trained personnel. Errors of diagnosis are fairly common. Many children do better on later tests than was originally expected.

4. Communication is a common problem, often compounded by the effects of other disabilities. Simplified sign systems or other means of non-speech communication may be necessary.

5. The behavior of multiply disabled deaf children is often misunderstood. In particular, caution is needed before concluding that a deaf child has a psychiatric disorder, a central language problem (aphasia), or mental retardation.

6. A developmental approach, with clearly specified objectives and frequent re-evaluation, is advisable as part of an educational program.

7. Schools for deaf children have an obligation to obtain better training for their staff to serve deaf children with additional disabilities; only in a centralized facility is it likely that there will be enough children to warrant such training.

8. Social circumstances may be at least as limiting as additional physical disability.

AFTERWORD

During the past year we exposed our ideas to over 60 experts. This resulted, as it should have, in an evolution in our thinking. We began with a bold ambition: to provide parents and professionals with a better awareness of choices concerning deafness by summarizing facts, opinions, and experiences and by reflecting fairly the weight of the evidence and of our own opinions, despite many uncertainties.

It has been painful to exclude much important information and illustrative material, some kindly provided by our resource people. The need to choose the most relevant material is proof that the field is now undergoing rapid change. Unfortunately we could not include our chapter on the history of deafness and of deaf people, because its length would have made the price of this book excessive, especially for parents. Although history *is* important, it is not likely to directly affect parental decisions, and the subject is covered elsewhere (Bender, 1970; Lane, 1979; Oyer, 1976). As a compromise, we offer to send the chapter (at cost) to anyone who requests it.

There have been many exciting developments in the field of deafness throughout the world. We realize that it has not been possible to do all of them full justice. If we have slighted any individual's or group's efforts, it is unintentional. A newly revised international listing of organizations and schools has just been published (Mathis, 1980). It may be helpful to those interested in contacts with other countries.

If we have any advice as a summary it is this: 1) uncertainties cannot be avoided, even when it would be more pleasant to pretend that an issue is settled; 2) professionals have an obligation to keep informed about new knowledge—often this responsibility is not taken as seriously as it should be; 3) the ways that deaf children and adults have found to live and succeed in a world that rarely understands them are remarkable and are worthy of study and respect; and 4) there is a great need for more and better research, especially long-range collaborative studies.

Responsible experimentation carries an obligation with it: to look unflinchingly at the possibility that *we might be wrong*, either totally or in part. Deaf people and their families have been subjected, and still are being subjected, to experimentation without their informed consent and without the kind of evaluation that should come from a blending of the scientific method with a humanistic spirit. This responsibility to be self-critical applies equally to all of us, regardless of our position on the methods controversy.

We have profound respect for all of those who helped us think more critically. Because of the very real disputes and differing values attached to deafness, it is inevitable that some readers will not be satisfied with our approach. If this is true of you, please tell us why so that the next edition may be improved.

If we have enabled parents to ask better questions and to feel that having a deaf child is not a tragedy, and if we have convinced professionals to consider more possibilities, we will have succeeded in ensuring, to some degree, that the lives of deaf children and the image of people who are deaf will be somewhat better in this uncertain world.

REFERENCES

Those references that we feel are intended for the general reader are marked with an asterisk (*). To aid those interested in purchasing some of the references, we have indicated those available from four of the major distributors as follows: (agba) = Alexander Graham Bell Association for the Deaf; (bda) = British Deaf Association; (gcb) = Gallaudet College Bookstore; and (nad) = National Association of the Deaf. (Addresses are listed in the section entitled "Resource List.")

Abrams, I. F. 1977. Nongenetic hearing losses. In: B. F. Jaffe (ed.), Hearing Loss in Children: A Comprehensive Text, pp. 367–375. University Park Press, Baltimore.

*Aldridge, L. D. 1980. Family Learning Vacation: An Implementation Guide. Special School of the Future, Gallaudet College, Washington, D.C.

Alexander Graham Bell Association for the Deaf. Undated, a. If Your Child is Deaf. The Association, Washington, D.C.

*Alexander Graham Bell Association for the Deaf. Undated, b. Listen! Hear! For Parents of Hearing-Impaired Children. The Association, Washington, D.C. (agba)

Altshuler, K. Z., Deming, W. E., Vollenweider, J., Rainer, J. D., and Tendler, R. 1976. Impulsivity and profound early deafness: A cross cultural inquiry. American Annals of the Deaf 121:331–345.

*Anonymous. 1974. A learning vacation. Gallaudet Today 5(1):6–11.

*Anonymous. 1979. Raising children. Monthly Letter, Bank Canadian National 10(7–8):1–4.

Arnold, D., and Tremblay, A. 1979. Interaction of deaf and hearing preschool children. Journal of Communication Disorders 12:245–251.

Baker, B. L. 1976. Parent involvement in programming for developmentally disabled children. In: L. L. Lloyd (ed.), Communication Assessment and Intervention Strategies, pp. 691–733. University Park Press, Baltimore.

Baker, C., and Battison, R. (eds.). 1980. Sign Language and the Deaf Community: Essays in Honor of William C. Stokoe. National Association of the Deaf, Silver Spring, Maryland.

*Baker, C., and Padden, C. 1978a. American Sign Language: A Look at its History, Structure, and Community. T. J. Publishers, Silver Spring, Maryland. (nad)

Baker, C., and Padden, C. 1978b. Focusing on the nonmanual components of American Sign Language. In: P. Siple (ed.), Understanding Language

Through Sign Language Research, pp. 27–57. Academic Press, Inc., New York.

Bartak, L., Rutter, M., and Cox, A. 1975. A comparative study of infantile autism and specific developmental receptive language disorder: I. The children. British Journal of Psychiatry 126:127–145.

*Batson, T. W., and Bergman, E. (eds.). 1976. The Deaf Experience: An Anthology of Literature By and About the Deaf. 2nd Ed. The Merriam-Eddy Co., South Waterford, Maine. (gcb)

Battison, R. 1978. Lexical Borrowing in American Sign Language. Linstok Press, Silver Spring, Maryland. (gcb)

Battison, R., and Jordan, I. K. 1980. Cross-cultural communication with foreign signers: Fact and fancy. In: W. C. Stokoe (ed.), Sign and Culture: A Reader for Students of American Sign Language, pp. 133–148. Linstok Press, Silver Spring, Maryland.

*Bender, R. E. 1970. The Conquest of Deafness (revised edition). Press of Case Western Reserve University, Cleveland/London. (gcb)

*Benderly, B. L. 1980. Dialogue of the deaf. Psychology Today 14(5):66–77 (October).

Bergman, A. B., and Stamm, S. J. 1967. The morbidity of cardiac nondisease in schoolchildren. New England Journal of Medicine 276:1008–1013.

Bergman, B. 1978. Current Developments in Sign Language Research in Sweden. British Deaf News, February Supplement. (bda)

Bergman, B. 1979. Signed Swedish. National Swedish Board of Education, Stockholm.

Bess, F. H. (ed.). 1977. Childhood Deafness: Causation, Assessment, and Management. Grune and Stratton, New York.

Biklen, D. 1974. Let Our Children Go: An Organizing Manual for Parents and Advocates. Human Policy Press, Syracuse, New York. (nad)

Blencowe, S. M. (ed.). 1969. Cerebral Palsy and the Young Child. Churchill Livingtone, Edinburgh/London (Longman Group, New York, 1971).

*de Bono, E. 1979. The Happiness Purpose. Penguin Books, Harmondsworth (U.K.)/Baltimore.

Bonvillian, J. D., Nelson, K. E., and Charrow, V. R. 1976. Languages and language-related skills in deaf and hearing children. Sign Language Studies 12:211–250.

Bornstein, H. 1979a. Sign language in the education of the deaf. In: I. M. Schlesinger and L. Namir (eds.), Sign Language of the Deaf: Psychological, Linguistic, and Sociological Perspectives, pp. 333–361. Academic Press, Inc., New York.

Bornstein, H. 1979b. Systems of sign. In: L. J. Bradford and W. G. Hardy (eds.), Hearing and Hearing Impairment, pp. 155–172. Grune and Stratton, New York.

*Bowe, F., and Sternberg, M. 1973. I'm Deaf Too: 12 Deaf Americans. National Association of the Deaf, Silver Spring, Maryland. (gcb, nad)

*Braddock, G. C. (author) and Crammatte, F. B. (ed.). 1975. Notable Deaf Persons. Gallaudet College Alumni Association, Washington, D.C. (gcb)

Brennan, M., and Colville, M. 1979. A British Sign Language research project. Sign Language Studies 24:253–272.

*Brill, R. G. 1978. Mainstreaming the Prelingually Deaf Child. Gallaudet College Press, Washington, D.C. (gcb, nad)

Brill, R. G., Merrill, E., Jr., and Frisina, D. R. 1973. Recommended Organizational Policies in the Education of the Deaf. Conference of Executives of American Schools for the Deaf, Washington, D.C.

*British Deaf Association. 1975. Gestuno. British Deaf Association, Carlisle, U.K. (World Federation of the Deaf international sign manual). (gcb, nad)

Bronfenbrenner, U. 1976. Is early intervention effective? Facts and principles of early intervention: A summary. In: A. M. Clarke and A. D. B. Clarke, Early Experience: Myth and Evidence, pp. 247–256. Open Books, London.

Brooks, P. H. 1978. Some speculations concerning deafness and learning to read. In: L. S. Liben (ed.), Deaf Children: Developmental Perspectives, pp. 87–101. Academic Press, Inc., New York.

*Browning, E. 1972. I Can't See What You're Saying. Paul Elek, London.

Bruch, H. 1954. Parent education or the illusion of omnipotence. American Journal of Orthopsychiatry 24:723–732.

Budden, S. S., Robinson, G. C., MacLean, C. D., and Cambon, K. G. 1974. Deafness in infants and preschool children: An analysis of etiology and associated handicaps. American Annals of the Deaf 119:387–395.

*Caccamise, F. 1978. New myths to replace old myths? American Annals of the Deaf 123:513–515.

Caccamise, F., Hatfield, N., and Brewer, L. 1978. Manual/simultaneous communication (M/SC) research. Results and implications. American Annals of the Deaf 123:803–823.

Caccamise, F., Dirst, R., DeVries, R. D., Heil, J., Kirchner, C., Kirchner, S., Rinaldi, A. M., and Stangarone, J. (eds.). 1980. Introduction to Interpreting for Interpreters/Transliterators, Hearing-Impaired Consumers, Hearing Consumers. Registry of Interpreters for the Deaf, Silver Spring, Maryland.

*Caley, R., and Gibson, L. 1978. Sex education and mental health. In: G. Montgomery (ed.), Of Sound and Mind: Deafness, Personality, and Mental Health; Papers Presented to the Scottish Workshop with the Deaf, pp. 39–45. Scottish Workshop Publications, Edinburgh.

*Carbin, C. F. 1976. A Total Communication approach: A new program for deaf infants and children and their families. British Columbia Medical Journal 18(5):141–142.

Castle, D. I. 1979. Telephone communication for the hearing impaired: Methods and equipment. Journal of the Academy of Rehabilitative Audiology 11(1):91–104.

Catlin, F. I. 1978. Etiology and pathology of hearing loss in children. In: F. N. Martin (ed.), Pediatric Audiology, pp. 3–34. Prentice-Hall, Inc., Englewood Cliffs, N.J.

Charrow, V. 1976. Manual English—A linguist's viewpoint. In: F. B. Crammatte and A. B. Crammatte (eds.), VII World Congress of the

Deaf (Proceedings), pp. 78–82. National Association of the Deaf, Silver Spring, Maryland. (gcb, nad)

Chasin, W. D. 1979. The clinical management of otologic disorders. In: L. J. Bradford and W. G. Hardy (eds.), Hearing and Hearing Impairment, pp. 93–108. Grune and Stratton, New York.

Chess, S. 1978. The plasticity of human development: Alternative pathways. Journal of the American Academy of Child Psychiatry 17:80–91.

Chess, S., Fernandez, P., and Korn, S. 1980. The handicapped child and his family: Consonance and dissonance, with special reference to deaf children. Journal of the American Academy of Child Psychiatry 19:56–67.

Chess, S., Korn, S., and Fernandez, P. 1971. Psychiatric Disorders of Children with Congenital Rubella, Brunner/Mazel, Inc., New York.

Cicourel, A. V., and Boese, R. J. 1972. Sign language acquisition and the teaching of deaf children. In: C. B. Cazden, V. P. John, and Dell Hymes (eds.), Functions of Language in the Classroom, pp. 32–62. Teacher's College Press, New York.

Clarke, B. R., and Ling, D. 1976. The effects of using cued speech: A follow-up study. Volta Review 78(1):23–34.

Cokely, D., and Baker, C. In press. American Sign Language: Student Texts. T. J. Publishers, Silver Spring, Maryland.

Connor, L. E. 1972. That the deaf may hear and speak. Volta Review 74:518–527.

Conrad, R. 1979. The Deaf Schoolchild: Language and Cognitive Function. Harper and Row, London. (gcb)

Conrad, R. 1980. Let the children choose. International Journal of Pediatric Otorhinolaryngology 1:317–329.

*Convention of American Instructors of the Deaf. 1980. Statement on P.L. 94–142. CAID Newsletter 10(8):1–2.

Cornett, O. 1967. Cued speech. American Annals of the Deaf 112:3–13.

Cornforth, A. R. T., Johnston, K., and Walker, M. 1976. The Revised Makaton Vocabulary. Royal Association in Aid of the Deaf and Dumb, London.

*Corson, H. J. 1976. Response to keynote address of Dr. R. J. Boese "The Preschool Years." In: F. B. Crammatte and A. B. Crammatte (eds.), VII World Congress of the World Federation of the Deaf (Proceedings), pp. 347–349. National Association of the Deaf, Silver Spring, Maryland. (gcb, nad)

Cotton, R. 1977. Progressive hearing losses. In: B. F. Jaffe (ed.), Hearing Loss in Children: A Comprehensive Text, pp. 482–489. University Park Press, Baltimore.

Council for Exceptional Children. 1980. Resolution: Least Restrictive Environment and Quality Educational Program for Exceptional Children (passed unanimously at April Delegate Assembly). CEC, Reston, Virginia.

*Craig, H. B., Sins, J. A., and Rossi, S. L. 1976a. Hearing Aids and You! Dormac, Inc., Beaverton, Oregon.

*Craig, H. B., Sins, J. A., and Rossi, S. L. 1976b. Your Child's Hearing Aid. Dormac, Inc., Beaverton, Oregon.

Critchley, M. 1975. Silent Language. Butterworths, London.

Cunningham, C., and Holt, K. S. 1977. Problems in diagnosis and management of children with cerebral palsy and deafness. Developmental Medicine and Child Neurology 19:479–484.

Dale, D. 1974. Language Development in Deaf and Partially Hearing Children. Charles C Thomas, Publisher, Springfield, Illinois.

Dale, P. S. 1976. Language Development: Structure and Function. 2nd Ed. Holt, Rinehart, and Winston, Inc., New York. (gcb)

Davis, H., and Silverman, S. R. 1978. Hearing and Deafness. 4th Ed. Holt, Rinehart, and Winston, Inc., New York, (gcb, nad)

*Davis, J. (ed.). 1977. Our Forgotten Children: Hard-of-Hearing Pupils in the Schools. National Support Systems Project and University of Minnesota Press, Minneapolis.

*Deafpride. 1976. Deafpride Papers: Perspectives and Options. Deafpride, Washington, D.C.

Deich, R. F., and Hodges, P. M. 1977. Language Without Speech. Souvenir Press, London.

Denmark, J. 1978. Early profound deafness and mental retardation. British Journal of Mental Subnormality 24 (Part 2, no. 47):1–9.

Denmark, J. C., Rodda, M., Abel, R. A., Skelton, U., Eldridge, R. W., Warren, F., and Gordon, A. 1979. A Word in Deaf Ears: A Study of Communication and Behavior in a Sample of 75 Deaf Adolescents. Royal National Institute for the Deaf, London.

*Denton, D. M. 1976. The philosophy of Total Communication. British Deaf News, August Supplement. (bda)

Deuchar, M. 1979. The grammar of British Sign Language. British Deaf News, June Supplement. (bda)

English, J. (ed.). 1978. Usher's Syndrome: The Personal, Social, and Emotional Implications. American Annals of the Deaf 123(3, May):357–422 (entire issue).

Erting, C. 1978. Language policy and deaf ethnicity in the United States. Sign Language Studies 19:139–152.

*Evans, L. 1977. Towards an effective education for deaf people in Britain. British Deaf News 11(1):2–3.

Evans, L. 1979. Psycholinguistic strategy for deaf children: The integration of oral and manual media. British Deaf News, February Supplement. (bda)

*Fairchild, B. 1979. Parental concerns. Journal of Rehabilitation of the Deaf 12:84–90.

*Farb, P. 1974. Word Play: What Happens When People Talk. (esp. pp. 157–187) Alfred Knopf, New York.

Farrugia, D., and Austin, G. F. 1980. A study of social-emotional adjustment patterns of hearing-impaired students in different educational settings. American Annals of the Deaf 125:535–541.

Farwell, R. M. 1976. Speech reading: A research review. American Annals of the Deaf 121:19–30.

*Fellendorf, G. W., and Harrow, I. 1970. Parent counselling 1961–1968. Volta Review 72:51–57.

Fenn, G., and Rowe, J. A. 1975. An experiment in manual communication. British Journal of Disorders of Communication 10(1):3–16.

*Finnie, N. R. 1975. Handling the Young Cerebral Palsied Child at Home. 2nd Ed. Heinemann, London (U.S. edition, Una Haynes, (ed.), published by E. P. Dutton and Company, Inc., New York.)

Fitch, J. L. 1972. Treatment of a case of cerebral palsy with hearing impairment. Journal of Speech and Hearing Disorders 37(3):373–378.

Fitz-Gerald, D., and Fitz-Gerald, M. 1976. Sex education survey of residential facilities for the deaf. American Annals of the Deaf 121:480–483.

Fraser, G. R. 1976. The Causes of Profound Deafness in Childhood. Johns Hopkins Press, Baltimore/Ballière and Tindall, London.

*Fraser, G. B. 1979. Genetic counseling in hearing impairment. In: A. T. Murphy (ed.), The Families of Hearing-Impaired Children, pp. 291–298. A. G. Bell Association for the Deaf, Washington, D.C. (Monograph issue of Volta Review 81(5), September). (agba)

*Freeman, P. 1975. Understanding the Deaf/Blind Child. Heinemann, London.

Freeman, R. D. 1967. The child psychiatric home visit: Its usefulness in diagnosis and training. Journal of the American Academy of Child Psychiatry 6:276–294.

Freeman, R. D. 1976. Some psychiatric reflections on the controversy over methods of communication in the life of the deaf. In: Royal National Institute for the Deaf, Methods of Communication Currently Used in the Education of Deaf Children, pp. 110–118. RNID, London.

Freeman, R. D. 1979. Psychosocial problems associated with childhood hearing impairment. In: L. J. Bradford and W. G. Hardy (eds.), Hearing and Hearing Impairment, pp. 405–415. Grune and Stratton, New York.

Freeman, R. D., Malkin, S. F., and Hastings, J. O. 1975. Psychosocial problems of deaf children and their families: A comparative study. American Annals of the Deaf 120:391–405.

Friedman, L. (ed.) 1977. On the Other Hand: New Perspectives on American Sign Language. Academic Press, Inc., New York. (gcb)

Fristoe, M., and Lloyd, L. L. 1978. A survey of the use of non-speech systems with the severely communication impaired. Mental Retardation 16(2):99–103.

Fulwiler, R. L., and Fouts, R. S. 1976. Acquisition of American Sign Language by a noncommunicating autistic child. Journal of Autism and Childhood Schizophrenia 6(1):43–51.

Fundudis, T., Kolvin, I., and Garside, R. F. (eds.). 1979. Speech Retarded and Deaf Children: Their Psychological Development. Academic Press, Inc., New York and London.

Furth, H. G. 1966. Thinking Without Language: Psychological Implications of Deafness. Free Press, New York/Collier-Macmillan, London. (gcb)

*Furth, H. G. 1973. Deafness and Learning: A Psychosocial Approach. Wadsworth, Belmont, California.

*Gallaudet College. 1975. What Every Person Should Know About Heredity and Deafness. Public Service Programs, Gallaudet College, Washington, D.C. ($0.50 U.S.) (gcb)

Gallaudet College. 1979. Directions, Vol. 1, no. 1 (entire issue on reading).

*Gannon, J. R. 1979. Shattering silence throughout the world. Presented at the Sixtieth Annual Convention of Quota International, July 16, Philadelphia, Pennsylvania.

*Gannon, J. R. 1980. Deaf Heritage: A Narrative History of Deaf America. National Association of the Deaf, Silver Spring, Maryland. (gcb, nad)

*Garretson, M. D. 1976. Total Communication. In: R. Frisina (ed.), A Bicentennial Monograph on Hearing Impairment, pp. 88–95. The Alexander Graham Bell Association for the Deaf, Washington, D.C. (agba, gcb)

*Garretson, M.D. 1977. The residential school. Deaf American 29(8):19–22.

Gath, A. 1978. Down's Syndrome and the Family: The Early Years. Academic Press, Inc., New York.

Givens, D. 1978. Social expressivity during the first year of life. Sign Language Studies 20:251–274.

Goldberg, J. P., and Bordman, M. B. 1975. The ESL approach to teaching English to hearing-impaired students. American Annals of the Deaf 120:22–27.

Goldin-Meadow, S., and Feldman, H. 1975. The creation of a communication system: A study of deaf children of hearing parents. Sign Language Studies 8:221–236.

Goodman, L., Wilson, P. S., and Bornstein, H. 1978. Results of a national survey of language programs in special education. Mental Retardation 16(2):104–106.

*Greenberg, J. 1970. In This Sign. Holt, Rinehart, and Winston, Inc., New York. (gcb, nad)

*Greenberg, J., and Doolittle, G. 1977. Can schools speak the language of the deaf? New York Times Magazine (December 11), pp. 50–52, 80–87, 90–102.

Greenberg, M. 1980a. Hearing families with deaf children: Stress and functioning as related to communication method. American Annals of the Deaf 125:1063–1071.

Greenberg, M. 1980b. Mode use in deaf children: The effects of communication method and communication competence. Applied Psycholinguistics 1:65–79.

Greenberg, M. 1980c. Social interaction between deaf preschoolers and their mothers: The effects of communication method and communication competence. Developmental Psychology 16:465–474.

Greenberg, M., and Marvin, R. S. 1979. Attachment patterns in profoundly deaf preschool children. Merrill-Palmer Quarterly 25:265–279.

*Gregory, S. 1976. The Deaf Child and His Family. Halsted, New York/ Allen and Unwin, London.

Haag, R. F. 1978. A residential program for deaf multi-handicapped children. American Annals of the Deaf 123:475–478.

*Hall, E. T. 1973. The Silent Language. Anchor Books, Garden City, New York.

Hammer, E. K. 1973. Deaf-blind clients: a behavioral model of rehabilitation services. Deafness Annual (Professional Rehabilitation Workers with the Adult Deaf) 3:15–29.

Harper, R. G., Wiens, A. N., and Matarazzo, J. D. 1978. Nonverbal

Communication: The State of the Art. John Wiley and Sons, Inc., New York.

Harris, R. I. 1978. Impulse control in deaf children: Research and clinical issues. In: L. S. Liben (ed.), Deaf Children: Developmental Perspectives, pp. 137–156. Academic Press, Inc., New York.

Hicks, W. M., and Pfau, G. S. 1979. Deaf-visually impaired persons: Incidence and services. American Annals of the Deaf 124:76–92.

Higgins, P. C. 1980. Outsiders in a Hearing World: A Sociology of Deafness. Sage Publications, Beverly Hills, California/London.

*Hockenhull, M. 1979. Enjoying life. British Deaf News 12(4):99–102.

Hoemann, H. W. 1975. American Sign Language: Lexical and Grammatical Notes with Translation Exercises. National Association of the Deaf, Silver Spring, Maryland. (gcb, nad)

Hoemann, H. W. 1979. Communicating with Deaf People: A Resource Manual for Teachers and Students of American Sign Language. University Park Press, Baltimore. (nad)

*Holcomb, R. 1977. The Hazards of Deafness. Joyce Media, Northridge, California. (gcb, nad)

Holmes, K. M., and Holmes, D. W. 1980. Signed and spoken language development in a hearing child of hearing parents. Sign Language Studies 28:239–254.

Holmes, L. B. 1977. Medical genetics. In: B. F. Jaffe (ed.), Hearing Loss in Children: A Comprehensive Text, pp. 253–265. University Park Press, Baltimore.

Ingram, R. M., and Ingram, B. L. (eds.). 1977. Hands Across the Sea: Proceedings of the First International Conference on Interpreting. Registry of Interpreters for the Deaf, Silver Spring, Maryland. (gcb, nad)

*International Association of Parents of the Deaf. 1976. Position statements (Introduction of Parents to Deafness; Total Communication; Total Family Involvement.) IAPD, Silver Spring, Maryland.

*International Association of Parents of the Deaf. 1979. Position Statements (Focus on Education; Public Law 94–142; Least Restrictive Environment; Child Evaluation and Placement; Individualized Education Program; Characteristics of an Appropriate Educational Program; Mainstreaming; Due Process). IAPD, Silver Spring, Maryland.

*Jacobs, L. M. 1974. A Deaf Adult Speaks Out. Gallaudet College Press, Washington, D.C. (Revised edition published 1980.) (gcb, nad)

Jan, J. E., Freeman, R. D., and Scott, E. P. 1977. Visual Impairment in Children and Adolescents. Grune and Stratton, New York.

Jensema, C. J., Karchmer, M. A., and Trybus, R. J. 1978. The Rated Speech Intelligibility of Hearing Impaired Children: Basic Relationships and a Detailed Analysis. Office of Demographic Studies, Series R, no. 6, Gallaudet College, Washington, D.C. (gcb)

Jensema, C. K. 1979. Communication methods used with deaf-blind children: Making the decision. American Annals of the Deaf 124:7–8.

*Jones, H. and Willis, L. 1972. Talking Hands: An Introduction to Communicating with People Who are Deaf. Stanley Paul, London.

Jordan, I. K., Gustason, G., and Rosen, R. 1979. An update on communication trends in programs for the deaf. American Annals of the Deaf 124:350–357.

*Jordan, J. M. 1971. "Doc, I can't hear so good." A deaf consumer views the medical profession. In: D. Hicks (ed.), Medical Aspects of Deafness (National Forum no. 4), pp. 14–18. Council of Organizations Serving the Deaf, Washington, D.C.

Kannapell, B. 1974. Bilingualism: A new direction in the education of the deaf. Deaf American 26(10):9–15 (also in Deafpride Papers: Perspectives and Options, 1976, pp. 43–50. Deafpride, Washington, D.C.)

Kannapell, B. 1978. Linguistics and sociolinguistic perspectives on sign systems for educating deaf children: Toward a true bilingual approach. Paper presented at the Second National Symposium on Sign Language Research and Teaching, October 16, San Diego, California.

Karchmer, M. A., and Trybus, R. J. 1977. Who Are the Deaf Children in Mainstream Education? Office of Demographic Studies, Series R, no. 4, Gallaudet College, Washington, D.C. (gcb)

Karchmer, M. A., Milone, M. N., Jr., and Wolk, S. 1979. Educational significance of hearing loss at three levels of severity. American Annals of the Deaf 124:97–109.

*Katz, L., Mathis, S. L., III, and Merrill, E. C., Jr. 1978. The Deaf Child in the Public Schools: A Handbook for Parents of Deaf Children. 2nd Ed. Interstate Printers and Publishers, Danville, Illinois. (gcb, nad)

Keane, W. M., Potsic, W. P., Rowe, L. D., and Konkle, D. F. 1979. Meningitis and hearing loss in children. Archives of Otolaryngology 105:39–44.

*Kelly, P. T. 1977. Dealing with Dilemma: A Manual for Genetic Counselors. Springer-Verlag, New York.

Klein, C. 1978. Variables to consider in developing and selecting services for deaf-blind children. Part 2. American Annals of the Deaf 123:430–433.

Klima, E., and Bellugi, U. 1979. The Signs of Language. Harvard University Press, Cambridge, Massachusetts. (gcb, nad)

*Knox, L. 1976. Parents' Perceptions. Bill Wilkerson Center, Nashville, Tennessee.

Konigsmark, E. W., and Gorlin, R. J. 1976. Genetic and Metabolic Deafness. Saunders, Philadelphia.

Kopchick, E. 1977. Mainstreaming deaf students using team teaching. American Annals of the Deaf 122:522–524.

Kyle, J. G., Jones, P. L., and Woll, B. 1979. The quality of interpreters. British Deaf News 12(3):62—63.

*Ladd, P. 1978. Communication or dummification: A consumer viewpoint. In: G. Montgomery (ed.), Of Sound and Mind: Deafness, Personality, and Mental Health; Papers Presented to the Scottish Workshop with the Deaf, pp. 46–51. Scottish Workshop Publications, Edinburgh.

*Lane, H. 1979. The Wild Boy of Aveyron. Harvard University Press, Cambridge, Massachusetts. (gcb, nad)

Lane, H. 1980. A chronology of the oppression of sign language in France and the United States. In: Lane, H., and Grosjean, F. (eds.), Recent Perspectives on American Sign Language, pp. 119–161. Lawrence Erlbaum Associates, Hillsdale, N.J.

*Lattin, D. 1975. Is this how a deaf person feels? Performance (President's Committee on Employment of the Handicapped), May, pp. 18–19.

Lennan, R. 1979. Factors in the educational placement of the multihandicapped hearing impaired child. In: E. H. Shroyer and D. Tweedie (eds.), Perspectives on the Multihandicapped Hearing Impaired Child (Monograph 2), pp. 23–31. Gallaudet College Press, Washington, D.C. (gcb)

Liben, L. S. (ed.) 1978. Deaf Children: Developmental Perspectives. Academic Press, Inc., New York.

von der Lieth, L. 1978. Social-psychological aspects of the use of sign language. In: I. M. Schlesinger and L. Namir (eds.), Sign Language of the Deaf: Psychological, Linguistic, and Sociological Perspectives, pp. 315–332. Academic Press, Inc., New York. (gcb)

Lindsey, D., and O'Neal, J. 1976. Static and dynamic balance skills of eight year old deaf and hearing children. American Annals of the Deaf 121:49–55.

Ling, D. 1978. Auditory coding and recoding: An analysis of auditory training procedures for hearing-impaired children. In: M. Ross and T. G. Giolas (eds.), Auditory Management of Hearing-Impaired Children: Principles and Prerequisites for Intervention, pp. 181–218. University Park Press, Baltimore.

Ling, D., and Ling, A. 1978. Aural Habilitation: The Foundations of Verbal Learning in Hearing-Impaired Children. The A. G. Bell Association, Washington, D.C. (agba, gcb)

Linthicum, F. H., Jr. 1979. New developments in surgery for hearing impairment. In: L. J. Bradford and W. G. Hardy (eds.), Hearing and Hearing Impairment, pp. 75–91. Grune and Stratton, New York.

Lloyd, L. I., and Kaplan, H. 1978. Audiometric Interpretation: A Manual of Basic Audiometry. University Park Press, Baltimore.

*Lowell, E. L. (ed.) 1976. Learning Steps: A Handbook for Persons Working with Deaf-Blind Children in Residential Settings. California State Department of Education, Sacramento.

*Luterman, D. 1979. Counseling Parents of Hearing-Impaired Children. Little, Brown and Co., Boston.

*McCormack, M. 1978. A Mentally Handicapped Child in the Family: A Guide for Parents. Constable, London.

McInnes, J. M., and Treffry, J. A. 1977. The deaf-blind child. In: Jan, J. E., Freeman, R.D., and Scott, E. P., Visual Impairment in Children and Adolescents, pp. 337–364. Grune and Stratton, New York.

*Mackey, P., and Heilman, J. R. 1978. "My deaf child leads a full life." Family Circle 91(8):46, 49–51, 150 (July 10).

Maestas y Moores. 1980. Early linguistic environment: Interactions of deaf parents with their infants. Sign Language Studies 26:1–13.

*Markowicz, H. 1977. Ameslan: Fact and Fancy. Public Service Programs, Gallaudet College, Washington, D.C. (nad)

Martin, F. N. (ed.). 1978. Pediatric Audiology. Prentice-Hall, Inc., Englewood Cliffs, N.J.

*Mathis, S. L. (ed.). 1980. International Directory of Services for the Deaf.

International Center on Deafness (Gallaudet College), Washington, D.C., and Interstate Printers and Publishers, Danville, Illinois.

Mayo, C., and La France, M. 1978. On the acquisition of nonverbal communication: A review. Merrill-Palmer Quarterly 24:213–227.

*Meadow, K. P. 1975. Subculture of the deaf. Hearing and Speech Action 43(4):16–18.

Meadow, K. P. 1979. The razor's edge: Working with parents of multiply handicapped children. In: E. H. Shroyer and D. Tweedie (eds.), Perspectives on the Multihandicapped Hearing Impaired Child (Monograph 2), pp. 1–10. Gallaudet College Press, Washington, D.C. (gcb)

Meadow, K. P. 1980. Deafness and Child Development. University of California Press, Berkeley.

Meadow, K. P., and Trybus, R. J. 1979. Behavioral and emotional problems of deaf children: An overview. In: L. J. Bradford and W. G. Hardy (eds.), Hearing and Hearing Impairment, pp. 395–403. Grune and Stratton, New York.

*Merrill, E. C., Jr. 1979. A deaf presence in education. British Deaf News, August Supplement. (bda)

*Miles, D. 1976. Gestures: Poetry in Sign Language by Dorothy Miles. Joyce Media, Northridge, California. (gcb, nad)

Mindel, E. 1971. Studies on the deaf child. In: R. R. Grinker (ed.), Psychiatric Diagnosis, Therapy, and Research on the Psychotic Deaf, pp. 73–83. Michael Reese Hospital and Medical Center (Chicago) and Social and Rehabilitation Service, Department of Health, Education, and Welfare (U.S. Government Printing Office), Washington, D.C.

*Mindel, E. D., and Vernon, M. 1971. They Grow in Silence: The Deaf Child and His Family. National Association of the Deaf, Silver Spring, Maryland (in revision, 1980). (gcb, nad)

Montgomery, G. 1976. Changing attitudes to communication: Some current trends in Scotland reviewed against recent international research and practice. British Deaf News, June Supplement. (bda)

Moores, D. F. 1978a. Current research and theory with the deaf: Educational implications. In: L. S. Liben (ed.), Deaf Children: Developmental Perspectives, pp. 173–193. Academic Press, Inc., New York.

Moores, D. F. 1978b. Educating the Deaf: Psychology, Principles, and Practices. Houghton Mifflin Company, Boston. (gcb, nad)

Moores, D.F., Weiss, K. L., and Goodwin, M. W. 1978. Early education programs for hearing impaired children: Major findings. American Annals of the Deaf 123:925–936.

Moores, D. F., Weiss, K. L., and Goodwin, M. 1981. Early Intervention Programs for Hearing Impaired Children: A Longitudinal Assessment. Gallaudet College Press, Washington, D.C. In press.

Moskowitz, B. A. 1978. The acquisition of language. Scientific American 239(5):92–108.

*Murkin, C., and Womersley, R. 1978. For Young Deaf People: A Guide to Everyday Living. Victorian School for Deaf Children (597 St. Kilda Rd.), Melbourne, Australia ($6.50 AUS).

Naiman, D. W. 1979. Educating severely handicapped deaf children. American Annals of the Deaf 124:381–396.

*Naiman, D., and Schein, J. D. 1978. For Parents of Deaf Children. National Association of the Deaf, Silver Spring, Maryland. (nad)

Naiman, D., Schein, J. D., and Stewart, L. 1973. New vistas for emotionally disturbed deaf children. American Annals of the Deaf 118:480–487.

Namir, L., and Schlesinger, I. M. 1978. The grammar of sign language. In: I. M. Schlesinger and L. Namir (eds.), Sign Language of the Deaf: Psychological, Linguistic, and Sociological Perspectives, pp. 97–140. Academic Press, Inc., New York. (gcb)

Nance, W. E., and Sweeney, A. 1975. Genetic factors in deafness of early life. Otolaryngologic Clinics of North America 8:19–48.

*National Foundation/March of Dimes. 1980. Genetic Counseling. The Foundation, Box 2000, White Plains, New York, 10602 (a public health education booklet available from the address given).

Nicholls, G. H. 1979. Cued Speech and the Reception of Spoken Language. Unpublished Master of Science Thesis, McGill University, Montreal.

*Nix, G. W. (ed.). 1977. The Rights of Hearing-Impaired Children. Volta Review 79(5) (entire issue). (agba)

*Nordén, K. 1978. Growing-up conditions for deaf children of deaf or hearing parents and hearing children of deaf parents. British Deaf News, February supplement. (bda)

Nordén, K. 1980. Learning processes and personality development in deaf children. Paper presented at the Third International Conference of the European Association of Special Education, August 4–8, Helsinki, Finland.

Nordén, K., and Ang, T. 1980. School placement of deaf and hard of hearing children. In: Research and Development Concerning Integration of Handicapped Pupils into the Ordinary School System, pp. 1–41. National Swedish Board of Education, Stockholm.

North Carolina Schools for the Deaf. 1979. Sex Education Curriculum. NCSD, Morganton, N.C.

Northcott, W. 1979. Guidelines for the preparation of oral interpreters: Support specialists for hearing-impaired individuals. Volta Review 81:133–145. (agba)

Northern, J. L., and Downs, M. P. 1978. Hearing in Children. 2nd Ed. Williams and Wilkins, Baltimore. (gcb)

*O'Rourke, T. J. 1978. A Basic Vocabulary: American Sign Language for Parents and Children. T. J. Publishers, Silver Spring, Maryland. (gcb, nad)

Oyer, H. J. (ed.). 1976. Communication for the Hearing Handicapped: An International Perspective. University Park Press, Baltimore.

*Pahz, J., and Pahz, C. 1977. Will Love Be Enough? A Deaf Child in the Family. National Association of the Deaf, Silver Spring, Maryland. (gcb, nad)

Pashayan, H. M., and Feingold, M. 1979. Heredity and deafness. In: L. J. Bradford and W. G. Hardy (eds.), Hearing and Hearing Impairment, pp. 125–144. Grune and Stratton, New York.

*Paul, M. E. 1973. Education as communication: Questions for educators of deaf persons. In: Deafpride Papers: Perspectives and Options, pp. 37–42. Deafpride, Washington, D.C.

Peckham, C. S., Martin, J. A. M., Marshall, W. C., and Dudgeon, J. A. 1979. Congenital rubella deafness: A preventable disease. Lancet i(8110):258–261 (February 3).

*Pfetzing, D. 1971. Diagnosis: Fact or fallacy. In: D. Hicks (ed.), Medical Aspects of Deafness (National Forum No. 4). pp. 67–70. Council of Organizations Serving the Deaf, Washington, D.C.

Porter, T. A. 1973. Hearing aids in a residential school. American Annals of the Deaf 118:31–33.

Power, D. J., and Quigley, S. P. 1971. Problems and Programs in the Education of Multiply Disabled Deaf Children. Institute for Research on Exceptional Children, University of Illinois, Urbana, Illinois.

Preisler, G. 1980. Modification of sign communication by a four year old deaf girl in four different settings. Paper presented at the Third Internation Conference of the European Association of Special Education, August 4–8, Helsinki, Finland.

Quigley, S. 1969. The Influence of Fingerspelling on the Development of Language, Communication, and Educational Achievement of Deaf Children. University of Illinois, Urbana, Illinois.

Rawlings, B., and Gentile, A. 1970. Additional Handicapping Conditions, Age at Onset of Hearing Loss, and Other Characteristics of Hearing Impaired Students, United States: 1968–69. Office of Demographic Studies, Gallaudet College, Washington, D.C. (gcb)

Rawlings, B. W., Biser, J. L., and Trybus, R. J. 1978. A Guide to College/Career Programs for Deaf Students 1978. Captioned Films for the Deaf Distribution Center and Gallaudet College, Washington, D.C.

Reich, C., Hambleton, D., and Houldin, B. K. 1977. The integration of hearing impaired children in regular classrooms. American Annals of the Deaf 122:534–543.

Reilly, J., and McIntire, M. L. 1980. American Sign Language and Pidgin Sign English: What's the difference? Sign Language Studies 27:151–192.

*Robinson, M. J. 1979. Sink or swim: The single-parent family with a deaf child. In: A. T. Murphy (ed.), The Families of Hearing-Impaired Children. The A. G. Bell Assn., Washington, D.C. (Monograph issue of the Volta Review 81(5):370–377, September). (agba)

*Rosen, R. 1979. A Parent's Guide to the Individualized Education Program (IEP). Gallaudet College Press, Washington, D.C. (gcb)

Ross, M. 1977. Hearing aids. In: B. F. Jaffe (ed.), Hearing Loss in Children, pp. 676–698. University Park Press, Baltimore.

Ross, M., and Giolas, T. G. (eds.). 1978. Auditory Management of Hearing-Impaired Children: Principles and Prerequisites for Intervention. University Park Press, Baltimore.

*Royal National Institute for the Deaf. 1976. Methods of Communication Currently Used in the Education of Deaf Children, RNID, London (2 vols.). (nad)

*Royal National Institute for the Deaf. 1978. Report of the Council of Management for the Year Ended 31st March 1978. RNID, London.

Rubin, M. 1979. Auditory training systems in perspective. In: L. J. Bradford and W. G. Hardy (eds.), Hearing and Hearing Impairment, pp. 193–205. Grune and Stratton, New York.

Rutter, M. 1980. School influences on children's behavior and development. Pediatrics 65:208–220.

Rutter, M., and Schopler, E. (eds.). 1978. Autism: A Reappraisal of Concepts and Treatment. Plenum Publishing Corp., New York.

Rutter, M., Maughan, B., Mortimore, P., and Ouston, J. 1979. Fifteen Thousand Hours: Secondary Schools and Their Effects on Children. Open Books, London.

Schein, J. D. 1968. The Deaf Community: Studies in the Social Psychology of Deafness. Gallaudet College Press, Washington, D.C. (gcb, nad)

Schein, J. D. (ed.). 1974. Education and Rehabilitation of Deaf Persons with Other Disabilities. Deafness Research and Training Center, New York University, New York City. (nad)

Schein, J. D. 1975. Deaf students with other disabilities. American Annals of the Deaf 120:92–99.

*Schein, J. D. 1977. Current priorities in deafness. Volta Review 79(3):162–174.

Schein, J. D. 1979a. Multiply handicapped hearing-impaired children. In: L. J. Bradford and W. G. Hardy (eds.), Hearing and Hearing Impairment, pp. 357–363. Grune and Stratton, New York.

Schein, J. D. 1979b. Society and culture of hearing-impaired people. In: L. J. Bradford and W. G. Hardy (eds.), Hearing and Hearing Impairment, pp. 479–487. Grune and Stratton, New York.

Schein, J. D., and Delk, M. T., Jr. 1974. The Deaf Population of the United States. National Association of the Deaf, Silver Spring, Maryland. (gcb, nad)

Schiefelbusch, R. L. (ed.). 1980. Nonspeech Language and Communication: Analysis and Intervention. University Park Press, Baltimore.

*Schlesinger, H. 1971. Prevention, diagnosis, and habilitation of deafness: A critical look. In: D. Hicks (ed.), Medical Aspects of Deafness (National Forum No. 4), pp. 19–30. Council of Organizations Serving the Deaf, Washington, D.C.

*Schlesinger, H. 1974. Diagnostic crises. In: P. M. Culton (ed.), Operation Tripod: Toward Rehabilitation Involvement by Parents of the Deaf, pp. 20–25. Pub. no. SRS 74–25020, U.S. Government Printing Office, Washington, D.C.

Schlesinger, H. S. 1978a. The acquisition of signed and spoken language. In: L. S. Liben (ed.), Deaf Children: Developmental Perspectives, pp. 69–85. Academic Press, Inc., New York.

Schlesinger, H. S. 1978b. The effects of deafness on childhood development: An Eriksonian perspective. In: L. S. Liben (ed.), Deaf Children: Developmental Perspectives, pp. 157–169. Academic Press, Inc., New York.

Schlesinger, H. S., and Meadow, K. P. 1972. Sound and Sign: Childhood Deafness and Mental Health. University of California Press, Berkeley. (gcb, nad)

Schlesinger, I. M., and Namir, L. (eds.), 1978. Sign Language of the Deaf: Psychological, Linguistic, and Sociological Perspectives. Academic Press, Inc., New York. (gcb)

*Schowe, B. M. 1979. Identity Crisis in Deafness. Scholars Press, Tempe, Arizona. (nad)

Schwirian, P. M. 1976. Effects of the presence of a hearing-impaired preschool child in the family on behavior patterns of older "normal" siblings. American Annals of the Deaf 121:373–380.

*Scott, E. P., Jan, J. E., and Freeman, R. D. 1977. Can't Your Child See? University Park Press, Baltimore.

*Selman, R. L., and Selman, A. P. 1979. Children's ideas about friendship: A new theory. Psychology Today 13(4):71, 72, 74, 79, 80, 114.

Shaffer, D., and Greenhill, L. 1979. A critical note on the predictive validity of "The Hyperkinetic Syndrome." Journal of Child Psychology and Psychiatry 20:61–72.

Shroyer, E. H., and Tweedie, D. (eds.). 1979. Perspectives on the Multihandicapped Hearing Impaired Child. (Monograph 2). Gallaudet College Press, Washington, D.C. (gcb)

Silverman, S. R. 1972. The education of deaf children. In: L. E. Travis (ed.), Handbook of Speech Pathology and Audiology, pp. 399–430. Appleton-Century-Crofts, New York.

Siple, P. 1978. Understanding Language Through Sign Language Research. Academic Press Inc., New York.

*Smith, L. 1973. Silence, Love, and Kids I Know. International Books, Washington, D.C. (nad)

*Smithdas, R. 1969. Life in My Fingertips. Doubleday and Company, Inc., New York.

*Spradley, T. S., and Spradley, J. P. 1978. Deaf Like Me. Random House, New York. (gcb, nad)

Stark, R. E. 1979. Speech of the hearing-impaired child. In: L. J. Bradford and W. G. Hardy (eds.), Hearing and Hearing Impairment, pp. 229–248. Grune and Stratton, New York.

Stevens, R. P. 1976. Children's language should be learned and not taught. Sign Language Studies 11:97–108.

*Stewart, L. G. 1974. We have met the enemy and he is us. American Annals of the Deaf 119:706–715.

Stewart, L. G. 1978. Hearing-impaired/developmentally disabled persons in the United States: Definitions, causes, effects, and prevalence estimates. American Annals of the Deaf 123:488–495.

Stokoe, W. C. 1978. Sign Language Structure: The First Linguistic Analysis of American Sign Language (revised edition). Linstok Press, Silver Spring, Maryland. (gcb)

Stokoe, W. C. 1980. The study and use of sign language. In: R. L. Schiefelbusch (ed.), Nonspeech Language and Communication: Analysis and Intervention, pp. 125–155. University Park Press, Baltimore (reprinted from Sign Language Studies 1976, 10:1–36).

Stokoe, W. C., Casterline, D. C., and Croneberg, C. G. 1976. A Dictionary of American Sign Language on Linguistic Principles (revised edition). Linstok Press, Silver Spring, Maryland. (gcb)

Terrace, H. S., Petitto, L. A., Sanders, R. J., and Bever, T. J. 1979. Can an ape create a sentence? Science 206 (4421):891–902.

Thomas, A., and Chess, S. 1980. The Dynamics of Psychological Development. Brunner/Mazel, Inc., New York.

Tibbenham, A. D., Peckham, C. S., and Gardiner, P. A. 1978. Vision screening in children tested at 7, 11, and 16 years. British Medical Journal i:1312–1314.

Topp, S. 1977. Abnormal central auditory processing. In: B. F. Jaffe (ed.), Hearing Loss in Children: A Comprehensive Text, pp. 490–501. University Park Press, Baltimore.

Trudgill, P. 1974. Sociolinguistics. Penguin Books, Harmondsworth, U.K./ Baltimore.

Tweedie, D., and Shroyer, E. H. (eds.). 1979. Hearing Impaired Mentally Retarded Children (Monograph 3). Gallaudet College Press, Washington, D.C. (gcb)

Tylor, E. B. 1871. Primitive Culture. John Murray, London (7th Ed., 1924, Brentano, New York).

van Uden, A. 1968. A World of Language for Deaf Children. Part 1: Basic Principles. St. Michielsgestel, The Netherlands (Rotterdam University Press).

van Uden, A. 1974. Religion and language in the pre-lingual deaf. In: D. H. Pokorny (ed.), My Eyes Are My Ears, pp. 231–242. MSS Information Corp., New York.

Vanderheiden, G. C., and Grilley, K. (eds.). 1977. Non-vocal Communication Techniques and Aids for the Severely Physically Handicapped. University Park Press, Baltimore.

Vernon, M. 1969. Multiply Handicapped Deaf Children: Medical, Educational and Psychological Considerations. Council for Exceptional Children, Washington, D.C. (nad)

*Vernon, M. 1975. Integration or mainstreaming (editorial). American Annals of the Deaf 120:15–16.

Vernon, M., and Koh, S. D. 1970. Effects of early manual communication on achievement of deaf children. American Annals of the Deaf 115:527–536.

Vernon, M., and Koh, S. D. 1971. Effects of oral preschool compared to early manual communication on education and communication in deaf children. American Annals of the Deaf 116:569–574.

*Vernon, M., and Makowsky, B. 1969. Deafness and minority group dynamics. Deaf American 21(11):3–6.

Vernon, M., Bair, R., and Lotz, S. 1979. Psychological evaluation and testing of children who are deaf-blind. School Psychology Digest 8(3):291–295.

*Watson, D. (ed.). 1973. Readings on Deafness. Deafness Research and Training Center, New York University, New York. (gcb, nad)

Wegner, D. M., and Vallacher, R. R. 1977. Implicit Psychology: An Introduction to Social Cognition. Oxford University Press, New York.

Wilbur, R. B. 1979. American Sign Language and Sign Systems. University Park Press, Baltimore. (nad)

*Wilson, E. A. 1976. Response to Dr. John Denmark: "Deafness and Mental Illness: The Rights of Deaf (Mental) Patients." In: Deafpride

Papers: Perspectives and Options, pp. 25–30. Deafpride, Washington, D.C.

Wong, D., and Shah, C. 1979. Identification of impaired hearing in early childhood. Canadian Medical Association Journal 121:529–546.

Woodward, J. 1979. Signs of Sexual Behavior: An Introduction to Some Sex-Related Vocabulary in American Sign Language. T. J. Publishers, Silver Spring, Maryland. (gcb)

Woodward, J. 1980. Signs of Drug Use: An Introduction to Drug and Alcohol Vocabulary in American Sign Language. T. J. Publishers, Silver Spring, Maryland.

Woodward, J. C., and Markowicz, H. 1980. Pidgin sign languages. In: W. C. Stokoe (ed.), Sign and Culture: A Reader for Students of American Sign Language, pp. 55–79. Linstok Press, Silver Spring, Maryland.

Wyke, M. A. (ed.). 1978. Developmental Dysphasia. Academic Press, Inc., New York and London.

*Yoken, C. 1979. Living With Deaf-Blindness: Nine Profiles. Gallaudet College Press, Washington, D.C. (gcb)

Zink, G. D. 1972. Hearing aids children wear: A longitudinal study of performance. Volta Review 74:41–51.

RESOURCE LIST

This list is far from complete. In particular, organizations serving deaf children with other disabilities are not listed. Those in your area can be contacted through local resources. An address is only given once for organizations and publishers. "Halex House" refers to the building shared by several organizations, located at 814 Thayer Ave., Silver Spring, Maryland 20910.

DISTRIBUTORS (OR PUBLISHERS) OF REFERENCES INDICATED IN THIS BOOK'S REFERENCE LIST (Each has a free catalogue):

Alexander Graham Bell Association for the Deaf, 3417 Volta Place, N.W., Washington, D.C. 20007 (*Volta Review*; International Parents' Organization—auditory/oral)

British Deaf Association, 38 Victoria Place, Carlisle, Cumbria CA1 1HU, U.K. (*British Deaf News*)

Gallaudet College Bookstore, Gallaudet College, Kendall Green, Washington, D.C. 20002 (also Division of Public Services; Gallaudet College Press; *Gallaudet Today, Directions*)

National Association of the Deaf, Halex House (*The Deaf American*)

OTHER PUBLISHERS:

Deafness Research and Training Center, New York University, 80 Washington Square East, New York, N.Y. 10003

Dormac, Inc., P.O. Box 752, Beaverton, Oregon 97005

Joyce Media, 8753 Shirley Ave., Northridge, California 91328

Linstok Press, 9306 Mintwood Street, Silver Spring, Maryland 20901

National Technical Institute for the Deaf, 1 Lomb Memorial Drive, Rochester, N.Y. 14623

T. J. Publishers, 817 Silver Spring Ave., Silver Spring, Maryland 20910

ORGANIZATIONS (selected periodicals in *italics*):

American Deafness and Rehabilitation Association, Halex House (*Journal of Rehabilitation of the Deaf*)

Association of Canadian Educators of the Hearing Impaired, 5 Duncan Crescent, Saskatoon, Saskatchewan S7H 4K3 (*ACEHI Journal*)

British Association of Teachers of the Deaf, 20 Devonshire Rd., Bolton BL1 4PJ, U.K. (*Teacher of the Deaf*; auditory/oral orientation)

British Deaf Association (*British Deaf News*)

Canadian Association of the Deaf, 2395 Bayview Ave., Willowdale, Ontario M2L 1A2

Canadian Coordinating Council on Deafness, 55 Parkdale Ave., Ottawa, Ontario K1Y 1E5 (*Communication*)

Conference of Educational Administrators Serving the Deaf, Halex House

Convention of American Instructors of the Deaf, Halex House

Deafpride, Inc., 2010 Rhode Island Ave., N.E., Washington, D.C. 20018

Gallaudet College (International Center on Deafness; Kendall Demonstration Elementary School; Model Secondary School for the Deaf; National Academy; Research Institute; Special School of the Future; and others)

International Association of Parents of the Deaf, Halex House (*The Endeavor*)

Junior National Association of the Deaf, c/o Gallaudet College (*The Junior Deaf American*)

National Association of the Deaf, Halex House (*The Deaf American*)

National Deaf Children's Society, 45 Hereford Rd., London W2 5AH, U.K. (*Talk*)

National Retinitis Pigmentosa Foundation, 8331 Mindale Circle, Baltimore, Maryland 21207

National Union of the Deaf, 3 Delaporte Close, Epsom, Surrey KT17 4AF, U.K.

Registry of Interpreters for the Deaf, Halex House

Royal National Institute for the Deaf, 105 Gower St., London WC1E 6AH, U.K. (*Hearing*)

Scottish Workshop With the Deaf, c/o Donaldson's School for the Deaf, West Coates, Edinburgh EH12 5JJ, U.K.

Telecommunications for the Deaf, Inc., Halex House

ADDITIONAL PERIODICALS:

American Annals of the Deaf, Halex House (the single most important journal for breadth of coverage)

Coup d'Oeuil, Centre d'Étude des Mouvements Sociaux, École des Hautes Études en Sciences Sociales, 54 Blvd. Raspail, 75270 Paris Cédex 06, France (excellent French journal on all aspects of sign language)

Cued Speech News, Gallaudet College, Cued Speech Programs

The Deaf Canadian c/o Deaf Canadian Readers' Assn., Box 1291, Edmonton, Alberta T5J 2M8

dsh Abstracts, c/o Speech-Language-Hearing Assn., 10801 Rockville Pike, Rockville, Md. 20852

Mental Health in Deafness, c/o St. Elizabeths Hospital, Washington, D.C. 20032

Sign Language Studies, Linstok Press
Signs for Our Times, c/o Linguistics Research Laboratory, Gallaudet College
Teaching English to the Deaf, c/o English Dept., Gallaudet College
Volta Review, A. G. Bell Association for the Deaf (auditory/oral)
The World Around You, Gallaudet College (magazine for deaf youth)

FURTHER READING

Since completing the text, the following important publications have come to our attention:

Benderly, B. L. 1980. Dancing Without Music: Deafness in America. Anchor/Doubleday, New York.

Bouvet, D. 1980. L'Enfant Sourd: Un Être de Langage. Monograph No. 20, Faculty of Psychology and Educational Science, University of Geneva, Switzerland.

Brennan, M., Colville, M. D., and Lawson, L. K. 1980. Words in Hand: A Structural Analysis of the Signs of British Sign Language. British Sign Language Research Project, Moray House, Edinburgh, U.K.

Chess, S., and Fernandez, P. 1980. Do deaf children have a typical personality? Journal of the American Academy of Child Psychiatry 19:654–664.

Chess, S., and Fernandez, P. 1981. The Handicapped Child in School: Behavior and Management. Brunner/Mazel, Inc., New York.

Fant, L. J., Jr. 1980. Intermediate Sign Language. Joyce Media, Northridge, California.

Federlin, T. 1979. A Comprehensive Bibliography on American Sign Language: A Resource Manual. Tom Federlin, 106 MacDougal St., New York, N.Y. 10012.

Humphries, T., Padden, C., and O'Rourke, T. J. 1980. A Basic Course in American Sign Language. T. J. Publishers, Silver Spring, Maryland.

Stelle, T. W. 1980. A Primer for Parents with Deaf Children: To Aid Understanding of Early Education and Communication. Scottish Workshop with the Deaf, Edinburgh. (Forty-two pages of sensible questions and answers.)

Stuckless, E. R. (ed.). 1980. Deafness and rubella: Infants in the 60s, adults in the 80s. American Annals of the Deaf, entire November issue, Volume 125, no. 8.

INDEX

Sign Languages—continued
  Siglish, 132, 133, 140, 156
  Signed English, 133
  Signed Swedish, 132
  Signing Exact English, 133
  Swedish Sign Language, 130,
    132
  technical sign development, 142
  theater, 139
  wit, 139
Simultaneous communication,
  154, 155
Single-parent families, 183
Smoke alarm, 287
Social relationships, 180–183
Social skills, 177, 181, 182
Sound conduction, 38, 39
Soundfield testing, 41
Southwest College for the Deaf,
  256
Soviet research, 208
Special education
  results, 149, 151
Speech
  cued, 117, 127, 128
  deaf, 114, 115
  diagnostic tests, 119
  intelligibility, 86, 87, 113, 115,
    245, 255
  internal, 115
  training, 5, 113–119, 158
Speech discrimination ability, 41
Speech range
  of hearing, 38
Speechreading, 84, 85, 87, 106,
    107, 116, 118, 127, 154,
    208
Speech reception threshold, 41
Speech therapy, 221

Stapes, 36
Syntax, 94

TDD, 282–286
Technical aids, 281–289
  wake-up alarms, 286
Telecommunication Devices for
  the Deaf, 282–286
Telephone
  use by deaf people, 281–286
Television
  captioned, 287
  special programs, 287–288
Temperamental patterns, 174,
    175, 300
Temper outbursts, 178
Threshold
  sound, 38
Tinnitus, 47
Total Communication, 85, 86,
    105, 147–164, 207, 222,
    225
Transliteration, 273, 274
TTY, 282
Tympanic membrane, 36
Tympanogram, 72

Usher's syndrome, 298, 299

Van Uden, Reverend Anthony, 18
Vertigo, 38
Visible English, 128, 133
Vision testing, 298
Visual impairment, 79, 238,
    296–299

Wake-up alarms, 286